Postpartum Depression and Anxiety

A self-help guide for mothers

Fourth Edition

PACIFIC POST PARTUM SUPPORT SOCIETY

First edition, 1987
Second edition, first printing, 1988
Second edition, second printing, 1990
Third edition, 1994
Third edition, in French, 1997
Fourth edition, 1997

Canadian Cataloguing in Publication Data:

Main entry under title:

Postpartum depression and anxiety : a self-help guide for mothers

4th ed.
Includes bibliographical references.
ISBN 0-9692983-2-3

1. Postpartum depression. I. Pacific Post Partum Support Society.

RG852.P68 1997 618.7'6 C97-901074-8

This book is dedicated to all the women who have shared their experiences with us. They have told us what it has been like for them and what has helped them. Their knowledge, wisdom and courage has made this book possible.

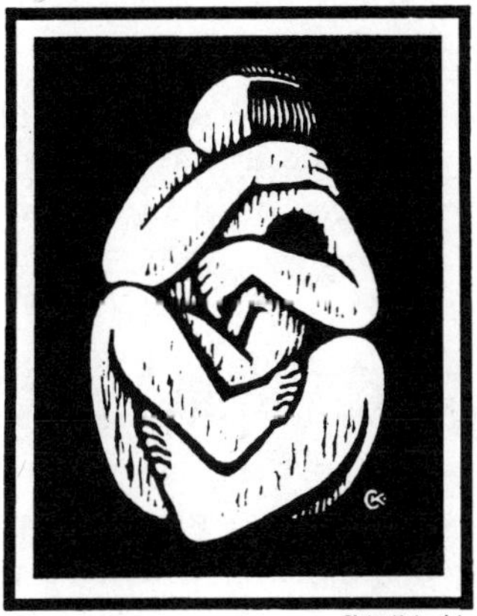

Claire Kujundzic

In order to broaden the scope of information and further document the range of women's experiences of postpartum depression for future editions of this book, we invite women of all cultures to write to us with new or different perspectives on postpartum depression.

Pacific Post Partum Support Society
1416 Commercial Drive, #104
Vancouver BC V5L 3X9
CANADA

1987 *Foreword*

At last! A book about postpartum depression which is sensible, practical, and informative. This is a book which stems from women's knowledge and wisdom, from the trials and tribulations of women's everyday lives, from the recognition of women's difficult and contradictory role in our society and their crucial but invisible and unrewarded work in the family. Medicine and psychiatry are stripped of their awesome and often unwarranted power and are demystified. Women's postpartum depression is clearly and logically shown to be related to stresses, strains, unrealistic expectations, cultural myths and images rather than being caused by genes, hormones or nasty childhood experiences.

This book celebrates women's strength in the face of tremendous adversity and almost impossible expectations. Under the circumstances it is amazing that only 20% of women become depressed. Instead of leaning on a medical or psychiatric formulation, thus putting the women in a sick role, this book empowers the depressed woman and helps her to engineer her own recovery. Instead of thinking that she is inadequate, neurotic, or even crazy, she gains understanding of her symptoms and is given strategies to begin to alleviate them. She learns to take time and space for herself, focus on her own needs, assert herself within the family and forge bonds with other women.

The timely birth of this book, the result of the labours of a group of dedicated women, will help dispel the secrecy, embarrassment and misunderstanding which still shrouds PPD and will allow many women to take charge of their lives.

Sue Penfold MB, FRCP(C),
Associate Professor in the Department of Psychiatry,
University of British Columbia
Child Psychiatrist,
British Columbia Children's Hospital

1997 *Foreword*

For women experiencing postpartum depression this *Self-Help Guide* is an essential first line aid. Before being offered counselling and medication, a woman with postpartum depression needs to know that she has not been struck by some unnameable, dark and irrational unhappiness just when she expected she would be enjoying one of the happiest experiences of her life. She has a well-known condition, the condition affects many others, it has universal features and universal causes, and there is help available for it. She is not alone.

The *Self-Help Guide* immediately helps to lift the burden of shame that afflicts a new mother with postpartum depression, the shame which is a hallmark of this experience and one of its first signs. "I have a beautiful baby and a wonderful husband, and I feel there must be something wrong with me if I can't be more happy," is the usual formulation of that shame. The very hearing of it should alert the health professional or friend to offer this guide. On opening it, the depressed mother will immediately find herself facing information and insight, empathetically presented, that provide a map both to her current troubled thoughts and feelings and to the paths leading back to wholeness and health. It is indispensible also to the father who himself is often bewildered and who has enormous difficulty hearing and understanding his partner's sense of desperation, fear, and isolation. It is being heard that is the first need of a woman with postpartum depression, and the very first step in the healing process.

This booklet hears attentively and it speaks with compassion and wisdom.

Gabor Maté, M.D.
Family Physician and Writer
Vancouver, British Columbia

Acknowledgements

Over the years, many people have worked together to create and update the *Self-Help Guide for Mothers.* The Pacific Post Partum Support Society especially wishes to acknowledge the following women, who wrote and organized the original edition of the *Guide*:

Penny Handford
Tricia Joel
Christine Bender
Nancy Ellard
Mary Hall
Lisa Parker-Jervis
and
Mona Reaume

We also thank Lee Saxell and Michelle LaRiviere, who worked on the book layout and contributed the graphics that were used in the first and all subsequent editions of the *Guide*, and Claire Kujundzic, who created the woodcut *Mother and Child* for the cover. This beautiful image became closely associated with the Pacific Post Partum Support Society and has been adopted as the Society's logo.

Thanks as well to Dr. Sue Penfold, Colleen Penrowley and the Vancouver Women's Health Collective, Dari and Dennis Rank, and Katherine Sample for their contributions to the original edition of the *Guide*.

We would also like to acknowledge the many people who contributed their time, energy and expertise to develop the second and third editions of the *Guide*, and also the French-language edition, *Angoisse et dépression post-partum – un guide pratique pour les mères.* For their work on these editions we thank Christine Bender, Marie Bourgeois, Julie Browne, Marie Geneviève Ceschi, Annie Ceschi, Denise de Montigny, Nancy Ellard, Clo Gilbert, Penny Handford, Jean Healey, Denise Hébert, Maureen Hogg, Tricia Hunter, Bill Hurst, Holly

Keller-Brohman, Linda King, Johanne Levesque, Hélène Lord, Ruth Makaroff, Sonya Makaroff, Mona Reaume, Anne Rosenberg, Nicki Sims-Jones, and Christine Villeneuve.

We thank, as well, Dr. Gabor Maté, who wrote the 1997 foreword to this, the fourth edition, and the following women who contributed new material and helped with revisions: Maureen Ainslie, Sheila Duffy, Sharon Flanagan, Clo Gilbert, Joy Hill, Tricia Hunter, Linda King, Shauna Little, Ruth Makaroff, Mona Reaume, Anne Rosenberg, and Alison Sales.

A very special thank-you goes to the family members of all of the above contributors to the *Guide.* This work would not be possible without their patience, encouragement and support.

The Pacific Post Partum Support Society is also very grateful to the organizations and departments of government that provided financial support for the various editions of this *Guide.* Thank you to Employment and Immigration Canada and the Vancouver Foundation for financing the development and printing of the first edition. Thank you again to the Vancouver Foundation, and to the United Church of Canada (Alma VanDusen Grant) for providing funds for printing the second edition. *Merci beaucoup* to the Regional Municipality of Ottawa-Carleton Health Department, our much appreciated partner in developing the French edition. We are also very grateful to Health Canada, Family and Child Health Unit, for their generous support for the development and printing of the French edition.

Finally, thank you to the many women who have written to tell us how the *Self-Help Guide* helped them through a difficult time. Their stories of struggle and recovery emphasize the need for increased awareness about the issues of postpartum adjustment and depression, and are an ongoing source of inspiration for the staff and volunteers at PPPSS.

The Pacific Post Partum Support Society
1997

Contents

Introduction

The idea for this book came from the realization that many women are suffering from some degree of postpartum depression and that very few will find access to supportive care while going through it. Some of our own mothers are only now feeling safe enough to talk about their experiences and describe how alone and crazy they felt.

The material in this book is based on over twenty-five years of counselling thousands of women with postpartum depression. These women have willingly shared their experiences with each other, and together they have explored what has helped them. It is their knowledge, wisdom, courage and generosity that has made this book possible. Emphasis has been put on those common threads which run through the experience of postpartum depression.

The book is divided into chapters with clearly marked sections so that you can easily find the information you need. There are many ways to read this book: by dipping into it and reading a small section; by reading it chapter by chapter in sequence; or by just reading those sections which interest you. You may come back to the book many times as different sections become relevant to your experience. Read this book in any way that feels right for you.

As you read, keep in mind that you are going to survive this. However hopeless you may feel, try to remember that it will end. Women grow and change as they cope with their depression. After it is all over, many women say they are glad they went through the experience. As one woman said, "I never thought I'd get through it but I did and I feel great. I know much more about myself. Now I enjoy my baby and I feel peaceful."

What is happening to me?

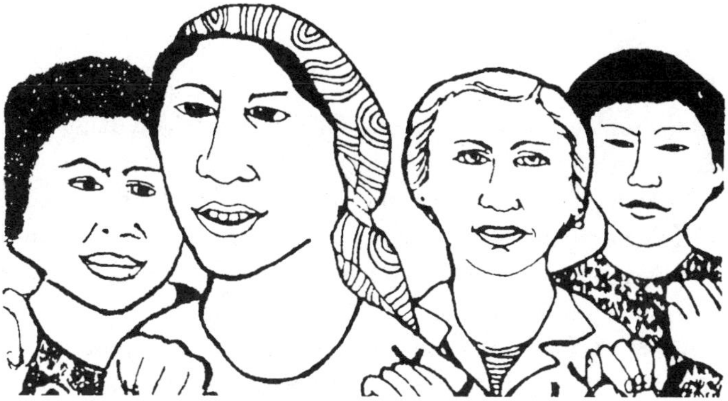

Most women expect to adjust easily to the arrival of their new baby. They anticipate feeling tired and somewhat disorganized, whether it is their first, second or sixth baby, but they still expect to feel good about themselves, their babies and families. For many women, however, this is not the case.

For 10-28% of mothers, the birth or adoption of a baby marks a change in their lives which is quite distressing. They may feel a range of emotions—from numbness and sadness to irritability, confusion and anxiety. Sometimes these feelings are accompanied by nightmares or scary thoughts. These experiences may begin soon after the arrival of the baby or many months later. They are usually very confusing and can be alarming to the woman and her family. If this is happening to you, you may be experiencing a postpartum depression. It is important for you to know that this is not uncommon—you are not going crazy and you are not a failure as a mother.

As a society, we place high expectations on motherhood, and often fail to understand when those expectations are not met. As a result, women find it difficult to talk about their depression. This leaves them silenced, lonely and isolated. We hope that this book will help to break this silence.

What is postpartum depression like?

Postpartum depression (PPD) can be described as "tearfulness, despondency, feelings of inadequacy and inability to cope".[1] It is more than a depressed mood, it continues for an extended period of time, and women definitely feel disabled by the experience. PPD is often accompanied by anxiety and overwhelming feelings of guilt, shame, isolation, fatigue, a sense of loss and, sometimes, very frightening fantasies.

Approximately one in five women experiences a postpartum depression. It is different from the "baby blues", which is a transitory tearfulness experienced by 80% of women on the third or fourth day after giving birth. PPD is also different from postpartum psychosis. Postpartum psychosis is very rare, affecting 0.1% of women and involving loss of contact with reality for extended periods of time.

The onset of postpartum depression may occur immediately after giving birth or many months later. The symptoms and experience of the mother during her depression are the same whether they occur at two weeks postpartum or after eighteen months. Moreover, the depression may occur after any birth, not necessarily only after that of the first child. The experience of the mother who becomes depressed after adopting a child is essentially the same. What follows are some feelings and experiences which are common during a postpartum depression.

"I am so irritable"

MOTHERS FEEL IRRITABLE and frustrated as an everyday part of raising young children. The intensity of these feelings may increase during a PPD. Many women talk about yelling at the older children, shaking the toddler, gritting their teeth, getting into screaming fights with their partners and generally being angry at themselves and the world. "As my body and mind became more and more exhausted I could hardly stand my baby crying, and there were moments when this sound was so painful that I was sure that I was going to hurt him if he didn't stop."

In view of the sadness, confusion and helplessness that many women experience, this anger and frustration is an understandable response. Sometimes women say it feels as if their anger could turn into a monstrous rage and they become anxious and frightened. Other women feel numb at this time; as they start to feel better, however, they get in touch with their anger and frustration. This may seem like a step backwards but, actually, it is a good sign, for it means that now they have the energy to feel their anger.

This frustration and anger can be a real surprise. Many find it hard to admit that they have resentful feelings towards those they love—the baby, the older children, their partner. It is really hard to say "I feel very angry at my baby". People generally do not understand this and may condemn the woman. Fearing such criticism, women often use words such as *upset* or *confused* and choose not to talk about these other feelings for fear of being labelled as a failure, unfit or abusive. There is nothing wrong with feeling angry but it is important to handle the anger safely. (See "Accepting the painful feelings" in the chapter "What helps?")

"I cry all the time" or "I feel like crying all the time but I can't"

IT IS VERY COMMON FOR women who are experiencing PPD to feel very sad or overwhelmed with emotion. Women talk about bursting into tears for no apparent reason, as if the tears come "out of nowhere". Other women say that they burst into tears when they watch certain commercials on T.V., hear a sad song or make a small mistake. "I just burst into tears at the slightest thing. I don't know what is happening to me." Many women think they may never stop crying—"It felt as if I would cry forever". On the other hand, some women feel very sad all the time but cannot cry. "I had a lump in my throat the whole time and my eyes hurt. I knew that if only I could cry I would feel better, but I couldn't."

It is very confusing and frightening for both the woman and her family when, instead of feeling happy after the arrival of the baby, she finds herself overwhelmed with sadness and emotion. They all need to know that this is a normal part of a postpartum depression and does not mean that she is "inadequate" or "a failure" or "unsuited to motherhood".

"I can't get going" or "I can't slow down"

WOMEN SEEM TO experience the depression and anxiety in different ways. Some have very little energy and look worn out and "untidy". They find it very difficult to make decisions and feel as if they are in a fog all the time. "I got to the point where getting dressed in the morning was too hard to do. I felt under tremendous pressure and I just couldn't handle it." Some will say, "I just can't move."

Other women, rather than being "slowed down", are full of nervous energy. Such "speedy" women are usually well groomed and seem to the outside world to be on top of things. Their house is usually tidy, they smile a lot and they are always busy. "I scrubbed, ran up and down stairs with a vacuum and generally did all I could so that everything seemed under control." Women who have this experience always have a list of jobs which need doing and can sometimes be seen at 2 a.m. ironing the laundry or cleaning the fridge.

Few people with whom the woman has contact realize how bad she is feeling because she puts up such a good "front". In fact, whether she outwardly appears slowed down or speedy, inside the woman is feeling miserable.

"I feel so worried all the time"

ANXIETY IS SOMETHING which often accompanies a postpartum depression. It may take the form of worrying about the health of the baby, other family members or oneself. Some mothers find themselves making frequent trips to the doctor or checking the baby's breathing at all times of day and night. "My nervousness made me lose milk and so the baby cried more often. My lack of control over the new situation left me frustrated. I felt like a failure and a sense of doom hung over me all the time."

Some women feel too anxious to stay at home alone and prefer to have other people around them. "When my husband left for work in the morning I would feel as if the walls were closing in around me. I felt trapped and whenever I could I left. I'd go to a friend's, to the shopping mall, anywhere, just so long as I could get out of the house." Others have the opposite experience and find themselves becoming agoraphobic. They find it very difficult to leave the house: for them, going to the shopping mall is a terrible ordeal. "I was terrified to go out the door and face people. If I did, I wouldn't know what to say, I'd sweat and stammer and make some excuse to rush away. Then I felt that they would talk about me behind my back. I really withdrew from people."

Housework and cleanliness are other common areas women may feel anxious about. "I just sit there and worry and worry about everything I have to do and it feels like I never get anything done." Others rush around compulsively cleaning and say such things as "I start doing the dishes before my husband has finished eating his supper".

Whichever way anxiety shows itself in a woman's life, it is commonly associated with postpartum depression.

"I am scared—I am having panic attacks"

SOME WOMEN EXPERIENCE "anxiety attacks" or "panic attacks". These have been described as any of the following: a pounding, racing heart, sweating or chills, shaking, hyperventilation, a choking sensation, chest pains, a sensation that one is about to black out, or a feeling that right at that moment, one is going crazy. These sensations are very frightening when they occur, and the woman may feel as if she is going to die. When she knows that they are, in fact, panic attacks, they are easier to cope with because even though they feel like they are going on for a long time they are generally short-lived.

"I can't feel anything"

SOME WOMEN REALIZE that there is something wrong because they feel numb. They don't feel sad or angry but they also don't feel happy, and have often lost their sense of humour. These mothers feel no close attachment or empathy for their babies. They say that they have "no feelings" for their babies. One woman said of her child, "She just didn't feel like my baby"; another said, "I expected to feel a flood of warm feelings when I looked at her. Instead I felt nothing." Sometimes the "numbness" creeps up on the woman gradually: "I enjoyed him in the hospital but for the last few weeks I have just felt numb". It is easy for the woman to start to feel crazy when she is receiving messages of congratulations and comments about how beautiful the baby is, and she is unable to feel any of this herself.

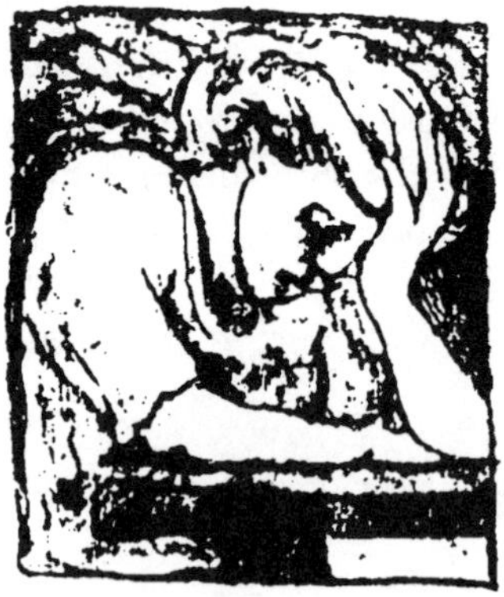

"I just can't cope"

WHETHER THE WOMAN is working from morning until night or can't get out of bed, she usually has a sense that it is impossible to do all the work which has to be done. It all seems meaningless and unending. There is also a sense that anyone could do the work better than she can. She usually blames herself for finding the work so difficult and may, in fact, be being blamed by others.

"I would lie in bed and say to myself—*You've got to be responsible and pull yourself together; no more of this childish nonsense.*" She may wonder, "How did I ever handle things before this baby was born?" She looks at her life and questions why she can't cope now. "I used to look after my toddler and go to work at the store. I managed everything then. I don't know what has happened to me since I had this baby." The whole experience takes on the quality of a nightmare. "I felt I was walking on a tightrope and that my nerves were going to snap. I tried to hide my feelings as much as I could. I was afraid to admit something was wrong. It all seemed like a bad dream."

"I feel so alone"

MOST WOMEN WHO ARE experiencing postpartum depression and anxiety think that "no one else has ever felt this way before". As a consequence of thinking they are "different" and failures as mothers, women often feel too embarrassed or ashamed to talk to each other about what they are really experiencing. Seeing other mothers chatting at the playground can be devastating for a depressed mother who feels incapable of joining in and wonders what's wrong with her. It seems as if she is the only one in the world who feels this way.

"I feel so guilty"

A WOMAN EXPERIENCING PPD blames herself and feels very guilty. She thinks that it's her fault she's doing so badly and causing so many problems for the family. "I feel so bad. I am not coping and everyone is worried about me." If the woman's partner is being supportive and doing the larger share of the household chores she feels like a burden. On the other hand, if her partner seems irritable and frustrated, the woman often thinks she's responsible for his moodiness.

The most intense guilt, however, is usually experienced around the baby and the older children. With all that is written about the importance of the first five years of a child's life, early bonding between the mother and child, and the effect of a stressful environment on children, most women are devastated by thoughts about the harm their depression might be doing. Often a vicious circle develops. Out of guilt about her depression, a mother may force herself to try and do more for her children than she's capable of. As a result, the woman's resentment and guilt increase. This makes her feel more depressed than ever.

"I feel so ashamed"

MOST WOMEN EXPERIENCING PPD feel ashamed. Even if they have heard about postpartum depression prior to experiencing it themselves, women are usually horrified by the nature of their feelings. "I am a terrible person, I have nothing to feel depressed about. I have a lovely baby, a wonderful husband, a nice home and yet I feel awful." This shame makes it very difficult for women to share their experiences until after their depression has passed. It keeps women who are experiencing postpartum depression isolated from each other and makes it very difficult for them to find the support they need. Some mothers are only now talking about the depression they experienced years ago.

"I don't know who I am any more"

ALMOST WITHOUT EXCEPTION, women who are experiencing PPD feel as if they have "lost" themselves. From being competent women, they feel as if they have become inadequate, helpless people.

All women have an image of what they will be like as mothers. Often things turn out very differently. A mother may have much less money than she expected, or end up parenting a child by herself when she believes children need both a mother and father in the family. Even if the circumstances are perfect, she may find that she is very disappointed by the experience of motherhood. Her image of herself as a mother is lost when she does not feel the way she expected after the arrival of the baby. "I always saw myself as a nurturing, caring mother who had time for the children. Instead I am tired, impatient and irritable—is this who I am?"

In the past she may have coped by taking time alone to sort things out. Now the demands of the baby prevent her from having any private time to do this. She struggles on, losing her sense of herself in the process. Some women say, "I don't know who I am. I don't know what to do. I feel as if I am in the middle of a windstorm being buffeted around." Others say, "I am walking through my chores like a robot. I know I don't want to be like this but I have no idea what I do want to be like."

Whether it is the first or fourth child, the identity crisis experienced by women after their baby is born is a major part of their depression.

"I can't sleep/ I want to sleep all the time"

SLEEP PATTERNS OFTEN change markedly during the postpartum period. Sleep deprivation and the broken sleep most women experience are major factors influencing energy levels and moods. Slowing down and relaxing enough to sleep can seem impossible. "I would lie awake at night and all the things I had to do, or I should have done differently, would run through my head." Many women can not get to sleep at all. "I was so tired but I couldn't sleep. I'd almost drop off, then something would snap in my head and that would set all my nerves jangling."

Other women find they can get to sleep initially but then wake up with frightening nightmares which leave them fearful of falling asleep. As the hours tick by, the woman may feel exhausted and overwhelmed at the thought of having to start a new day. "It seemed like an endless cycle. I'd go to bed thinking—*if I can only sleep, tomorrow will be better.* As dawn would approach, I would feel hopeless at the thought of dragging through another day." Lack of sleep caused by insomnia or a wakeful baby or both can cause severe anxiety and increase the woman's stress load.

Conversely, some women use sleep as a means of escape and each morning is a struggle to get up. "My two year old would join me in bed when she awoke around 9 a.m. I remember her tiny fingers prying at my eyelids, and her asking me for food. I would plead, 'Let mommy sleep a few minutes more'."

Some women spend the day dozing, getting up only to look after their children's basic needs or when their partner is due home. "I would lie on the couch, my baby on my chest and go in and out of sleep—getting up only when she needed attention. Every time I got up I felt disgusted with myself and how little I was doing. I longed to go back to sleep so I wouldn't have to think or feel." The lack of energy becomes more serious with an older, more active baby or child, as they require constant supervision.

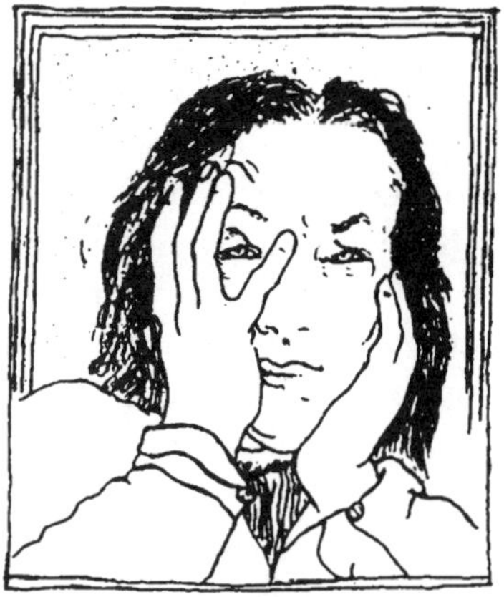

"I feel so ugly"

AFTER A WOMAN HAS a baby, she usually weighs more than before the pregnancy. Her muscle tone may be poor, and her breasts are often swollen with milk. Her body can feel very strange and out of her control. It takes some effort and perseverance to get back into shape. When a woman is feeling anxious and depressed she may not have the energy or time to take care of her body.

If a woman has put a great deal of emphasis on her physical appearance this experience can be devastating. As one woman said, "What was especially debilitating was the feeling that my body had fallen apart."

"I can't stop eating/I don't want to eat"

OVEREATING AND MILD anorexia are common symptoms when a woman is going through a postpartum depression. Some women eat compulsively. "I couldn't pass the cookie jar without taking one. It was the only comfort I got." This can lead to the added stress of putting on weight and feeling out of control and ugly. Sometimes a woman's feelings or beliefs about breastfeeding can add to this stress. "My body somehow seemed no longer my own. I felt that, in order to nurse my baby, I should eat well. Losing weight was therefore impossible, and I had little control over my body and how it looked."

Other women don't want to eat when they are feeling down, or they simply forget. They may feel anxious or speedy, and think that they have no time to stop to eat. They will cook for their family but find that, after the children have eaten, there is usually no time for their own meal.

"I don't want sex any more"

MANY WOMEN SEEM TO lose all interest in sexual contact at this time. When a woman is going through a PPD she usually feels tired, tense and overwhelmed, as well as ugly and uncomfortable with her body. She may also be frightened of becoming pregnant again.

This lack of sexual interest can cause a lot of guilt and anxiety about whether sexual feelings will ever return, and it can put a strain on the relationship. On the other hand, some women have found that their partners withdraw from them and they feel confused and rejected. Usually, both men and women feel nervous about discussing their decreased sexual interest with each other, even though it is extremely common for sexual activity to decrease when there are young children.

"I am having very scary thoughts"

IT IS VERY COMMON for women who are experiencing PPD to have frightening fantasies. The fantasies can be thoughts, visual images, sounds or voices.

Fantasies of harming the child are common—"I really love him but I imagined myself throwing him out of the window". These fantasies increase the feelings of guilt, shame, and worthlessness. "I wished that by some miracle I'd wake up to find that it was all a horrible dream. I feel so badly about the thoughts I have." Sometimes a woman can become so terrified by the thoughts she is having of hurting her child that, in an attempt to control the thoughts, she will turn them inward and fantasize about hurting herself. This serves to increase the intensity and frequency of her fantasies, heightening her anxiety.

Sometimes the woman is haunted by painful memories. These memories are described by the mother as "coming out of the blue" and "having a life of their own". Often she does not realize until later, as her depression lifts, that they are in fact memories—"I used to see sudden pictures of blood. I was terrified. I thought that it meant that I was going to hurt someone. It wasn't until I felt better that I realized that these were memories of something I had seen when I was young".

When women experiencing postpartum depression have scary thoughts, they usually feel as if they are going crazy. This is not the case. These fantasies are commonly experienced when a woman is going through a postpartum depression.

Why me?

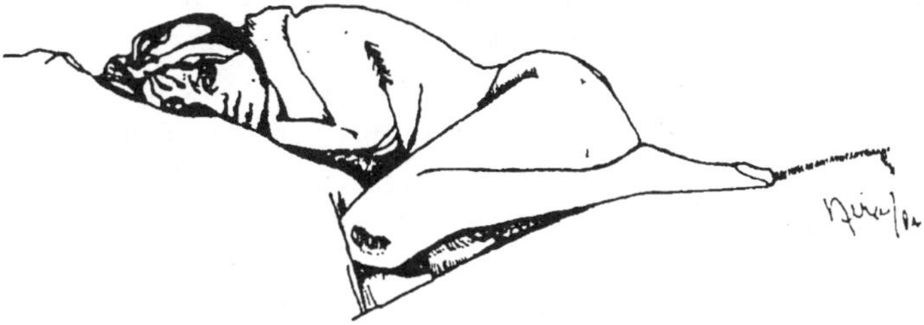

When a woman realizes that she is feeling down, she expects to feel better soon. But when she is experiencing a postpartum depression, she does not feel better quickly. Even if she does, it lasts for only a few days and then she feels down again. If she is fortunate, when she realizes something is wrong either she or someone else will identify that what she is going through is a postpartum depression. Her first thought will often be *Why me?*

At this point, many women search for the "cause" of their depression, believing that if they can understand the cause, they will be able to take control of their lives again. However, postpartum depression is not caused by one single thing and, for individual women, contributing factors will vary; postpartum depression must be looked at in a multidimensional way. Unfortunately, there are no simple explanations or quick solutions.

This chapter discusses factors which may be contributing to the postpartum depression, although no one factor will ever be the sole reason a woman is experiencing PPD.

"Is it my hormones?"

SOME THEORIES HOLD that the dramatic reduction of the mother's estrogen and progesterone occurring after birth is the cause of the depression.[2] Some women are undoubtedly more sensitive to hormonal changes than others. Indeed it may be that the hormonal swing does cause some women to become depressed postpartum. However, this does not account for the many women who become depressed many months after the birth. This seems to be clearly stress-related, as does the depression experienced by women who adopt children. Interestingly, there seems to be a hormonal change which occurs when men and women are in high stress situations. The hormonal changes after birth are apparently similar to those experienced by people in combat.[3] It could be a question of which comes first, the chicken or the egg.

"Did I get depressed because of my birth experience?"

IT SEEMS TO SOME women that the traumatic nature of the birth experience itself causes their depression. Most women plan their labour and delivery very carefully. They attend childbirth preparation classes with their partner or friend and plan to be supported by that person during delivery. Some women develop birth plans and may employ a midwife. Most women, although nervous, eagerly anticipate the birth.

Too often, however, the birth experience is a disappointment, even for women who did not plan in great detail. Some women feel that they were treated with little respect in the hospital and that they had no control over what happened to them.

Other women have difficult births. The baby might be premature or there might have been some other problem. The woman may end up reluctantly taking drugs or having a C-Section. When things do not go as planned, it can be very confusing for the mother. She may be left wondering if the medical intervention was really necessary, or if she agreed to surgery too quickly. She may feel that she was not assertive enough with the medical staff. Even though it is not her fault, she often blames herself for what happened. She can feel violated and abused by the experience. When things do not go well, the woman often feels like a failure and experiences a great sense of loss and disappointment.

Some women have unhappy birth experiences and develop a depression. Others have similar experiences and do not. Some women have "perfect" home births and still feel depressed. The nature of the birth may be a factor in the woman's postpartum depression and it may be something that causes her a lot of pain and distress, but it is never the single issue which causes the depression.

"Is it because I have a difficult baby?"

SOME WOMEN FEEL that they are depressed because their baby is particularly difficult to cope with. The baby may be premature and spend time in the hospital after the mother comes home. The baby may be sick or colicky or may just fuss for no apparent reason. Alternatively, the baby may sleep a lot, causing the woman to fear that there is something wrong with her child.

It is very stressful when a woman considers her baby to be "difficult" for any reason whatsoever. There is no doubt that lack of sleep, frustration and anxiety about the baby's health can contribute to a postpartum depression. However, a particular problem is only one of many factors contributing to PPD. For example, the woman will often find that even when the colic (or whatever) has gone away, she still feels depressed.

"Is it because I'm breastfeeding?"

SOME WOMEN THINK, or are told, that their depression is related to the fact that they are breastfeeding, and they quit in the belief that this will cure the depression. It rarely does.

Some women with PPD say that nursing is the one time they feel close to the baby and good about being a mother. They may feel that breastfeeding is the one thing they can do well for the baby. In that case, breastfeeding may be a source of comfort for the mother.

However, breastfeeding can also be very stressful. The nursing mother is physically tied to her baby in ways in which a mother who is bottle feeding her baby is not. Breastfeeding can feel like an extension of pregnancy with the woman feeling that her body is not her own. When a woman is nursing, it can be very hard for her to get time for herself. If a woman feels depressed and desperately needs time away, breastfeeding can be another source of stress.

Also, when a baby is having trouble sucking or when a mother is having difficulty with her "let-down reflex", the "failure" of the breastfeeding can seem like more "proof" that the woman is an inadequate mother.

Breastfeeding is not a cause of postpartum depression. The decision whether or not to nurse is a very personal one which each woman has to make for herself.

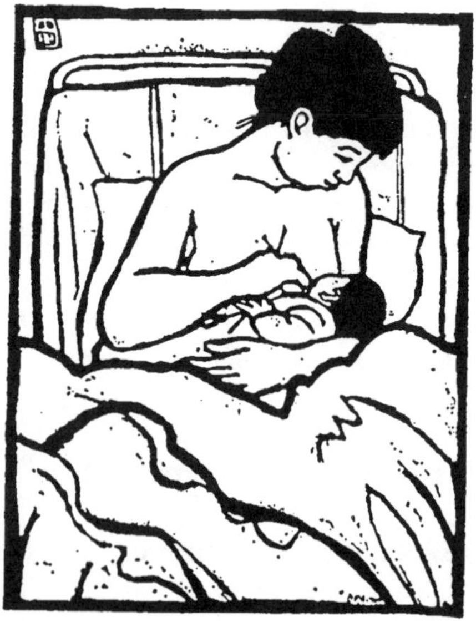

"Maybe I had the baby at the wrong time"

WHEN OLDER WOMEN become postpartum depressed, they often question their decision to have had children later in life, saying "Nobody told me it would be like this—I looked forward to my new life with this lovely baby for so long and now I don't know if I can cope". Younger women are afraid all the messages received from society are true: "You are too immature to cope with the demands of a small baby". Both groups of women need a lot of reassurance that women of all ages get postpartum depression and that it is not a reflection of their ages.

Financial problems can also cause many women to feel that the baby came at the wrong time. Financial stress definitely can add to a PPD but there is no correlation between financial status and PPD. "I thought as soon as I had money coming in everything would be fine. It was a shock to return to work and end up feeling worse."

"Is it because of my past?"

PREGNANCY AND CHILDBIRTH are times of tremendous changes. Many issues from the past such as family relationships and painful events come to the surface. For some, this is the time when memories of things that happened in childhood resurface. Women who were physically or sexually abused or both as a child may find themselves reliving the feelings they had at the time of the abuse. This is very painful and each woman needs as much support as possible, especially from other women who have survived similar traumas. While recognizing the effects of these in a postpartum depression, it is important to see the factors in the present situation as well. There are numerous aspects of the life of a mother of young children that contribute to the distress.

What helps?

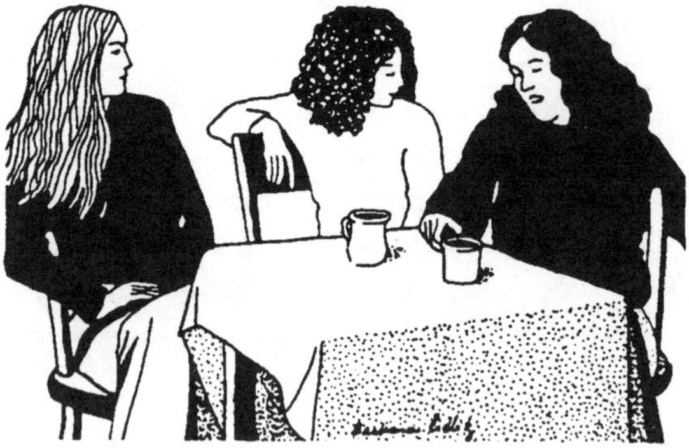

The most important thing a woman with PPD needs is to talk, in confidence, with other mothers who have had the same experience. Through this, women discover that their feelings are similar, regardless of the differing details of their situations.

Sometimes women take a drug such as an antidepressant or tranquilizer in the hope that it will make them feel better. Such drugs may lessen or even eliminate the symptoms of depression, but it may take several weeks before they provide relief, and some women do not respond to them at all. Other women experience distressing side effects that drugs can cause, and may eventually decide to taper off their medication (with their doctor's help). (See the chapter "Medications—making an informed choice".) Also, these medications do not deal with the stressors that may have triggered the depression. For these reasons, women need to do other things to help them resolve their depression, even if they have started taking medication.

This chapter contains suggestions which many women have found useful. When you are reading these sections, it's important to distinguish between short- and long-term goals. In the long term you might need to get a sitter and other helpers to come in once a week so that you can get regular breaks. This will take a lot of time and effort. Your short-term goal may be to get a small break today by sitting down for a few minutes while the children are sleeping or watching T.V. It is important that you do small things to help yourself immediately, and as you feel a little better you will be able to take steps to reach your long-term goals.

You will probably need to read this chapter many times as you go through your PPD. A suggestion which does not seem to apply to you when you first read it may do so later, because as time goes on your needs may change. What follows are some things which women have found helpful in regaining a sense of themselves and of control over their lives.

Nurturing yourself

EVEN IF YOU THINK YOU are not getting anything done, remember that care of a baby and small children requires an immense amount of work. It may seem impossible to get any time for yourself. You may find yourself taking care of your baby, your partner and your family, either by constantly cooking, cleaning and doing the laundry or by sitting and worrying about doing them. In either case, none of your energy is being used to take care of yourself. You deserve nurturing too. Nobody can be expected to give to others twenty-four hours a day without also giving something to herself.

The idea of getting time for yourself probably seems overwhelming. You can start by taking small amounts of time—even five minutes to sit down and have a cup of tea can help. Some ideas of ways that women have found to nurture themselves are taking a bubble bath, buying a bunch of flowers, having coffee with a friend or reading a magazine. Whatever comes to mind that you have not found time for is probably what's right for you. It has to be something you like to do, not something you think you should do.

Nurturing yourself also involves treating your emotional needs with respect. When you feel sad and lonely you might need to take care of these feelings by getting a hug, wrapping yourself in a blanket or curling up on the couch. It may help if you can find a small, comfortable space in your home that you can call your own. This could be a favourite chair by the window or a corner of your bedroom which is pleasing to you.

Getting a break

BEFORE YOU CAN EVEN think about what you need, it is necessary to have some time for yourself. Somewhere, during each day, you deserve at least one break from mothering—maybe a leisurely bath when the baby is asleep. Your need for a break is much more important than doing the housework. After all, when you have a paid job you get coffee and lunch breaks, and often you don't work as hard as you do as a mother!

When you are a mother working at home what you really need is the chance to leave the house without the children—either alone or with your partner. Making the move to leave your baby with someone else is a big step, yet essential as a way of establishing your right to some time to yourself.

Don't be discouraged if you don't feel free to enjoy yourself the first time and find yourself worrying whether everything's all right. Most of us did exactly the same and it will get easier.

Single parents may find it particularly difficult to organize breaks. For the most part, they live on low incomes with no extra money to pay for child care. Moreover, building a network of people to care for your child takes a lot of work and energy. For many single parents, small breaks at home while their children are occupied are the only breaks they get.

When you are a woman working outside the home, getting time for yourself can be very difficult. When you have been away from your children all day it can be hard to justify taking more time away. You may feel that going to work is a break from your children, but it is still important to make time just for you.

Finding child care

FINDING SOMEONE TO trust with your children may seem an enormous task and you may wonder where to start looking. It might seem easier just to keep the kids with you all of the time. But the hard work of finding someone will pay off in the long run, and you will feel better for the break.

Breaking down the process into small steps and completing one step at a time usually makes it more manageable. You will probably feel anxious about leaving your child with someone else the first few times. If you can, stay at home with your babysitter until you feel comfortable leaving, then leave for a little while. You will probably feel guilty at first, but find that after the first few times it's easier to enjoy yourself.

It may happen that you find child care that seems appropriate to you but is unacceptable to your partner. If this happens several times it may be because your partner is having some difficulty with the idea. In this situation, you may need some support to assert your right for time away from the children. It is important to talk openly with your partner about this.

Single mothers, as well as women who have less money to pay for a sitter, often have to rely on each other for child care. However, taking care of other children may take energy that you don't feel you have right now. This is why it is important to keep on looking for a reliable child care provider in order to get a regular break.

Take advantage of any community centre activities or parents' support groups with child care provided. Other resources might include established child care services in the community. Some of these services may have subsidies for low income families.

Some ideas of where to find child care providers include the following:

- Local newspaper (you might want to put your own ad in)
- Health clinic
- Local high school (talk to counsellor)
- Community centre
- Church groups
- Friends, neighbours, relatives, their teenage children
- Local child care support programs or child care resource centres. These kinds of organizations, as well as your health department, often provide a detailed guide you can follow in choosing safe, quality child care.

What about sleep?

SLEEP CAN BE A MAJOR issue in a postpartum depression. If you find yourself sleeping all the time, reassure yourself that this is your body's coping mechanism. You're not lazy. This is just one way of handling pain and stress for a time. Be gentle with yourself. As you work through your depression your energy will gradually return.

If you are having difficulty sleeping at night, lying down to rest during the day can help revitalize your body even if you don't sleep. Look at your day and plan times when you can rest. Whenever your baby is sleeping, rest instead of doing housework.

The most important thing you can do to help yourself at night time is to develop a routine which enables you to slow down and relax before you go to bed. For example, a useful routine might be to have a bath, lie on the couch to read for a few minutes and then go to bed.

The following suggestions may be helpful for general relaxation and getting to sleep:

- Take a brisk walk in the fresh air
- Drink a glass of warm milk and honey
- Write down all your plans and/or worries
- Have a candle-lit bath with no interruptions
- Reduce the amount of caffeine in your diet

Medication is commonly prescribed for sleeping difficulties. Many women have found that they can reduce or eliminate the need for medication by following the suggestions made here. If you have a prescription please refer to the chapter on medications, "Medications—making an informed choice", for further information on their use.

Accepting the painful feelings

ACCEPTING THE PAINFUL feelings can be very difficult, especially if you are frightened by what is happening. You may think that because you are experiencing sadness, irritation, resentment, frustration or rage, you are a bad person or unsuited to mothering. If you are not used to these feelings it can be difficult to believe that they are not abnormal. They are just feelings, however, and they are not going to destroy you.

Crying a great deal does not mean that you are a weak person. Tears can be healing and actually relieve stress. Even though it feels as though the tears will never end, they will stop when they have run their course. You might find yourself thinking of many different things when you are crying, such as the horrible birth experience you had or how much you miss your job. You may have no idea why you are crying. Sometimes when you cry, you find yourself thinking of things you haven't thought about in years. You may cry about a long-forgotten hurt or you may find yourself grieving for a loss from which you thought you had recovered. In all cases, the important thing is to give your sadness time. If possible let someone you trust hold you while you cry. Let yourself cry as much and as deeply as you can for as long as you need.

If what you feel is a lot of irritation and frustration, you may think that you are going to be a bitter, angry woman for the rest of your life. A common response to this is to try to push down these unpleasant feelings. But censoring them has the opposite effect because it usually prolongs the feelings. What helps is to air your angry feelings. This means giving yourself permission to get angry in a safe way without taking it out on another person or hurting yourself.

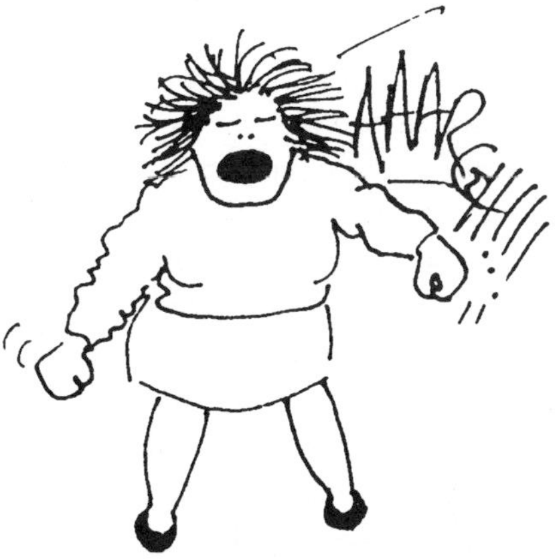

Anger can range from mild irritation, resentment or frustration, to profound rage. It is important that you find the outlet which works best for you. What works one day may not work a week later, so it is important to develop a range of different ways of coping with the anger. The following are some suggestions:

- Scream into a pillow
- Pound a pillow, a counter or a table
- Scream in the shower or in the car
- Tear up magazines, papers, old sheets
- Run up and down stairs
- Skip rope
- Break something that doesn't matter (put it in a bag so that you don't have to clean up)
- Write a letter expressing your anger but don't mail it
- Keep a journal of your feelings
- Draw angry pictures
- Hit the side of the bath tub with a towel
- Wring a towel
- Bite a towel

If you find yourself feeling angry while holding the baby, put the baby in the crib and try one of the above suggestions.

It is not easy to do these things; you will probably feel silly when you first try them. However, it is much better for you to release your anger in one of these safe ways than to take it out on your children or partner.

It can take some time before you start feeling better. Generally these techniques do not work the first time. You have to do them regularly as there is often a backlog of anger to deal with.

Many women feel very anxious about physically expressing their anger. Women have been taught that this is not appropriate behaviour for them. However, releasing anger from your body by using your large muscles can be very empowering. Sometimes, though, this seems impossible, especially if you have grown up in a family which was physically abusive. If so, try writing angry letters, drawing angry pictures or anything else that works.

Your partner may be scared of your anger, especially if he is not comfortable with his own. He may make it difficult for you to express your anger. He might think that you are going crazy.

It depends very much on how comfortable he is with emotions. You will need to be very clear with him that what you are doing is an appropriate way of dealing with anger and stress. If it is still an issue for him, you might choose to do it alone in the bathroom or bedroom with the door closed.

Accepting your anger and finding a safe way to express it is difficult and demanding work, but it is one of the most important things you can do to help yourself get better.

Dealing with fantasies

THE VIVID FANTASIES which can go with postpartum depression can be terrifying. Usually they start to go away as the woman starts to feel better, but while they are present it is necessary to develop coping strategies.

The most important thing to remember is that these fantasies are just images. They can be visual or auditory and can feel very real but they are NOT real. They usually tend to become worse at night or when you are tired. Generally speaking, they also become worse the more stressed you are. When you have a scary thought, remind yourself that the thought is not the same as the action and does not have to be acted out. Thinking of harming the baby does not mean you actually will harm the baby. Picturing yourself driving the car over a cliff does not mean that you will do it.

When you can, it usually helps to get away from the children when you are having a scary fantasy. Put the baby down in a safe place and go into another room. There you could try deep breathing or skipping on the spot, or having a good cry or whatever helps to relieve the tension and clear your head. Do not try to control these thoughts by trying to make them stop. Fighting the fantasies just makes you more anxious and this in turn will make you have more fantasies.

Some women have vivid images of knives and blood. If you are experiencing anything like this, you may feel better if you take some action such as putting the knives away in a safe place, or getting someone else to hide them for you. Doing this helps, not because you are likely to do harm, but because you will feel safer and calmer when the knives are out of sight. When you feel better you can get them out again.

Sometimes the scary thoughts are actually horrible memories from when you were a child. For example, if you were sexually abused, you may find yourself reliving it and suddenly seeing pictures in your mind of yourself, or maybe your child, being violated. Another example would be that, if you watched your father physically abuse your mother when you were small, you may see vivid images of this in your mind when you are going through a postpartum depression. If this is happening to you, it might be appropriate to seek out a counsellor to talk about the confusion you are experiencing. You might have to work through the memories of the abuse before you can recover from the postpartum depression.

Whatever type of fantasies or scary thoughts you are having, it will always help to talk to a supportive friend about them. However, if you find that your friend becomes scared when you tell her, she might not be the one to talk to. You need someone who is comfortable enough when hearing your fantasies to give you the reassurance that you are not going crazy. Unfortunately, many people, including some doctors and psychiatrists, become nervous on hearing about fantasies and therefore cannot be supportive. You may wish to call one of the organizations listed in the chapter "Resources" if you cannot find someone locally you can talk to about fantasies.

Finally, some other suggestions for dealing with frightening thoughts and fantasies include ways of addressing the thoughts directly. You could pretend the fantasy is on tape and cut up the tape. You could imagine a huge eraser wiping out the fantasy. Using your imagination to fight the thoughts can be a very effective tool. Try always to remember that the fantasies are only thoughts and feelings which arise because you are in a very stressful situation right now. They are a common part of a postpartum depression and do not mean that you are going crazy.

Coping with suicidal thoughts and feelings

THE SUICIDAL THOUGHTS and feelings experienced during a postpartum depression are very frightening. They range from the occasional thought, to frequent powerful fantasies, to actually planning to commit suicide.

It is important to try not to ignore the way you are feeling. Although having such thoughts does not mean you are going to kill yourself, it is important to take these thoughts seriously and take good care of yourself. Trying to ignore the thoughts and feelings will make things worse—you will get tense and more depressed. Accepting that something is wrong, and looking for ways to take care of yourself, will help. You must put your own needs first at this time.

When you start to feel better the suicidal thoughts go away. But while they are present it is necessary to develop coping strategies. It helps to get the thoughts out in the open: tell someone you can trust, or call a crisis line or a suicide prevention centre.

When you have a suicidal thought, try to stop what you are doing (put the baby down in a safe place); do some deep breathing; punch a pillow; go for a walk or jog. If you are driving, pull over to the side of the road, open the window, take some deep breaths and do something routine like combing your hair.

When the thought or feeling has passed, try to see if anything triggered it. Have you been rushing around without a break for days? Are you overtired? Has something happened which felt like the final straw? Have you had a painful memory? It is important to put your suicidal feelings in the context of your life so that you can understand them.

If you find yourself seriously making plans of how you can kill yourself, you must tell someone. For example, if you find yourself saving pills, it is important to call someone who can help you plan ways to cope, such as a mental health centre or crisis line.

Suicidal feelings are not unusual during a postpartum depression. It is understandable to want to escape the pain. Sometimes it feels as if the pain will never end. It does.

Paying attention to the good feelings

WHEN YOU ARE GOING through a postpartum depression, it is important to pay attention to those times when you feel a little better. Something may make you smile or you may have a pleasant memory. You may be feeling generally "numbed out" around your baby, and yet you may notice she has a sweet smile or soft silky hair. Try to pay attention to these moments, no matter how fleeting. Do not dismiss them. This is not the same as what is generally called "positive thinking", which can imply pushing away painful feelings and superimposing a cheerful facade. Instead, it means noticing and cultivating genuine feelings of love and pleasure when they arise.

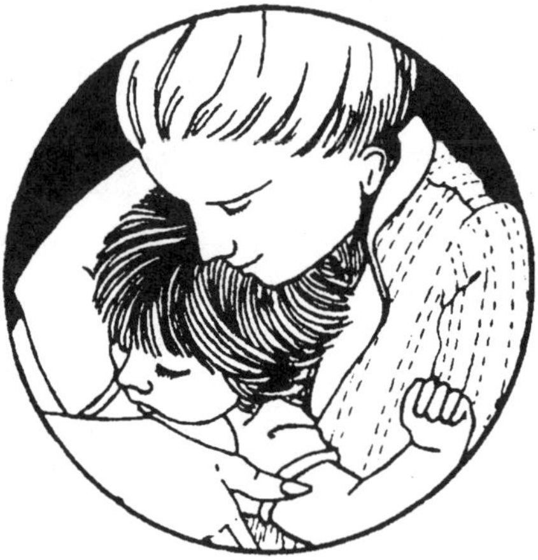

Taking one step at a time

WHEN SOMETHING LOOKS overwhelming it usually helps to break it down into small steps. When you feel like you can't get anything done, choose one task to complete within the next seven days. If you've got too much to do, cut your list for today in half.

If you can never sit still, try sitting down and breathing deeply for a moment, then gradually increase the length of time you are able to rest. Should getting out of the house seem impossible, start by opening the door and standing on the porch for a short time. If you surpass your initial goal, consider the extra accomplishment a bonus.

Doing something physical

THE IDEA OF PHYSICAL exercise can be quite tedious or intimidating to some women. It might remind them of school physical education classes and they immediately resist the notion. If you are feeling low and have no energy, the idea may seem impossible. It is important that getting some exercise does not become another "should" on your list of things to do. You can begin with thinking about what you'd like to do. It's not necessary to jog or play racquetball: a simple walk is beneficial. It leaves you relaxed and more in touch with your body, and it helps to clear your head. Joining an exercise group can be fun, as you may meet other women, and child care is often provided.

Eating as well as you can

WOMEN ARE BOMBARDED daily by messages pressuring them to diet and look thin. A woman in the postpartum period is more vulnerable to this pressure as she's frequently uncomfortable with how her body has changed because of the pregnancy and birth.

When a woman is depressed, she often either overeats or feels that she cannot eat at all. If you are having problems with overeating it is important that you do not blame yourself. You will find that as you feel better you will eat better. It may take a long time for your body to become stabilized, and it's not good to lose weight rapidly during this time. If you are breastfeeding, you have to consume a lot more calories than you normally would. It's not appropriate to go on any crash diets. If you are having problems eating anything at all, don't force yourself to eat when you can't. When you feel like eating, pay attention to what your body wants and eat that.

It is a good idea to have basic, easy-to-eat nutritious foods in your fridge. If you have cheese, fresh fruit, peanut butter, yogurt and raw vegetables easily accessible, you will tend to snack on them. It is also a good idea to have whole grain bread, nuts, dried fruits and other such things in your cupboard. Most important of all, try to listen to what your body is telling you.

Some women have found Vitamin B supplements to be useful. Others say a multivitamin helped. If you are not eating very well or very nutritiously, you might consider taking some vitamins, but consult your doctor first. Inform your doctor in any case if you have concerns about your diet.

Keeping your expectations realistic

IN OUR SOCIETY, very high expectations are placed upon mothers. They are supposed to be nurturing, supportive, calm, contented people who are fulfilled by caring for others. Family members usually look to the mother to be the emotional "caretaker". She is expected to mediate in disputes, pacify upset children, solve conflicts and generally take care of the family's emotional welfare.

Most women incorporate these expectations into their self-image and expect to be a calm, nurturing caregiver under all circumstances. These expectations are unrealistic. Inevitably, women cannot live up to them and then feel very critical of themselves.

If this is happening to you, you probably feel irritable and resentful. You may take great pride in your housekeeping and feel like a failure when your house is a mess, even though it is not reasonable to keep your house spotless when you have a baby or small children. At this time, it is very important to examine your expectations. Are they realistic in your circumstances or are you pushing yourself too hard? Where did the expectations come from? From family members or from messages you received as a child about what a "good" mother is? When you have identified the expectations you are putting on yourself (and possibly the sources), you can begin the process of lowering your expectations of yourself, or perhaps even letting some go.

High expectations of oneself usually lead to high expectations of others. You may expect your two year old to behave in ways which are unrealistic for such a young child. When the child can not meet your standards you may feel like a failure as a mother. As you start to lower these expectations of yourself, you will become more accepting both of your own limitations and those of others.

Coping with anxiety attacks

HAVING AN ANXIETY or panic attack can be a very frightening experience. You can feel as if you are having a heart attack or "going crazy". A panic attack is a physiological reaction to stress. It is harmless and will pass.

If you are having anxiety attacks, you have two things to think about: first, how to reduce your level of stress and take better care of yourself and, second, how to manage the attack when it is occurring. Some techniques to try that many women have used to get through anxiety attacks include the following:

- focus on breathing
- take a distracting action such as combing your hair
- talk with someone about what is happening
- visualize pleasant experiences.

After a panic attack it is common to feel very tired. Rest for a while.

As long-term strategies, many women find that dealing with their angry feelings (see "Accepting the painful feelings" in this chapter) and taking breaks are most effective in helping to alleviate the panic attacks.

Developing a support system

DEVELOPING A SUPPORT SYSTEM is an important part of recovery. You will find that people can help you in many ways: by encouraging you to nurture yourself; by assisting you, step-by-step, to accomplish difficult tasks; by supporting you in decisions you make; by acknowledging the work you do. People in your support system can be a resource for practical information or assistance—or they can be there just to listen.

As you begin to reach out and make contact with other people, don't be discouraged if you find your first few attempts do not work out. It takes time to find out if someone can support you in the way you want. Also, don't expect to have all your needs met by one person. You'll probably find that some needs are met in one place and some in another.

Many women look for support in places such as women's centres, family places, babysitting co-ops, and moms' and tots' groups. People you may want to include in your support system are neighbours, friends, public health nurses, family members, family doctors and counsellors.

Some women find support in a postpartum depression support group. One of the most healing aspects of attending a support group is hearing other women in the group talk about the sad, angry, scary feelings that each of them has been experiencing. Most women find it a tremendous relief to realize that they are not alone in feeling this way. They also find it inspiring to hear how other women make changes in their lives, and to see the growth that occurs as a woman resolves her depression and moves on from the group.

There are other places, besides support groups, where you can find caring support from someone who understands. For instance, after recovering from PPD, many women want to help others who are going through the experience. Sometimes they volunteer to support a mother over the telephone. You might be able to arrange such support through your doctor, public health nurse, a local postpartum support program, or one of the organizations listed in the chapter "Resources" at the back of this book. You can also receive caring, understanding support from professional practitioners who are knowledgeable about PPD.

The chapter "Getting help from professional helpers" lists some questions to bear in mind when you are looking for a doctor, psychiatrist or therapist; some of these questions may also be useful when seeking support from non-professional helpers or when thinking of attending a particular support group.

Wherever you find someone who can give you support, it is a good idea for each of you to clearly understand the other's needs and expectations. If appropriate, you may wish to give your helper this book to read, especially the chapter "How the helper can help".

Your helper, for her part, will need you to understand when and how often she can give you support. She may be available on short notice, or she may arrange to support you at certain times during the week. Either way, sometimes she may tell you that "right now is not a good time". In that case, you can arrange a time that would be better. You may feel that you need her support right then, but she will be less able to help you if she is feeling uncomfortable.

If finding a good time becomes a recurring problem, or if your helper seems resentful or irritable, she may be overextending herself. If that is the case, she will need to take some time to care for herself. This does not mean that she is abandoning you or that now you must take care of her. It simply means that, for a while, she will not be able to give you support. If you have more than one person supporting you, this situation is less likely to occur.

As you build up your support system, you will find that it becomes easier to make changes in your life and to acquire skills that will help you to recover. A good support system takes work to develop, but is well worth the time and effort you put into it. It evolves as your needs change, and its benefits last a lifetime.

Getting through it—will it ever end?

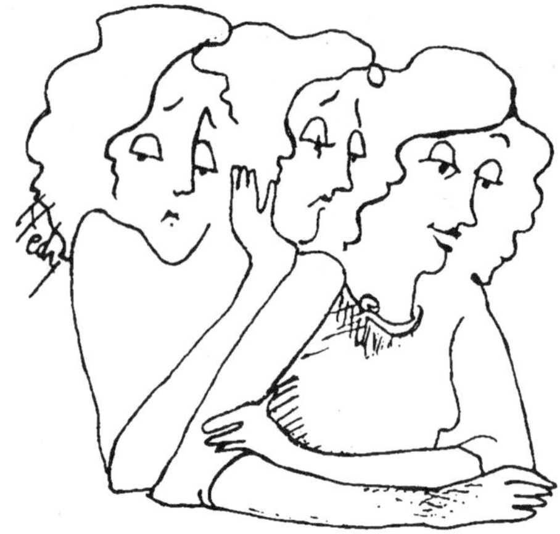

The process of recovery is different for each woman. For one woman the first step may be to find five minutes to sit down and rest. For another, it might be to get out of a housecoat and into some clothes. Whatever your circumstances, getting through this experience is not easy. It takes a lot of patience, perseverance and courage.

At first you will probably think that the suggestions in the chapter "What helps?" seem rather trivial. You may think that sitting down for five minutes is useless; what you really need is two weeks in bed. Of course you are right. You do need more than five minutes rest. However, you CAN arrange a five-minute break, while you probably can't arrange a two week vacation right now, and in the long run, the five minutes you DO get will make the difference. You may also think that the suggestions in the chapter "What helps?" about finding safe ways to deal with your frustration and anger are a bit silly. Hitting a pillow may seem pointless, or you may feel uncomfortable because you've been told that expressing anger is childish, weak or out of control. Many women have felt that these suggestions will not work.

It is important that you know that they have worked for thousands of women. They will work for you, if you keep on trying.

It is especially difficult if you are struggling through this alone. You may not feel better right away after you start to take care of yourself. You may even feel worse for a while. As you allow yourself to get in touch with your feelings of sadness and anger, you may feel that you are becoming more depressed. Try not to panic. What is happening is that you are becoming aware of painful feelings that have existed all along. For some women the sequence of events was that, at first, they cried all the time, then they felt numb and finally they got in touch with their feelings and found themselves feeling sad and angry. If this happens to you, when you find yourself crying again, your first reaction will probably be *Oh no—I'm back to square one!* It feels like that, but you are not going backward, nor will you cry forever, even though it feels like it sometimes. Your tears will take their own course and will be healing, actually helping to relieve the stress.

It might help at this time to talk to a trusted friend about these feelings. Maybe you could ask her to read this book so that she can understand what is happening to you. What is important is that even though the feelings are very painful, you are not going crazy and you will survive. Expressing the feelings in confidence to someone you trust will help, as will taking breaks, and doing all the little things you can do each day to take care of yourself.

For a while (maybe a few weeks), you may feel as if you are taking two steps forward and one step back. When you start to get a break for yourself you will probably find that after all the hard work it took to arrange, you feel too guilty to enjoy it, or you'll have a relaxed time away from the family but as soon as you walk back into the house you want to turn around and walk out again. You may feel angrier after you have had a break than you did before. Sometimes it feels as if you are getting nowhere.

What is happening, however, is that you are finding out how things work for you and getting in touch with your real feelings. It is also a time when you are becoming realistic about the expectations you put on yourself. Gradually you will start to get an understanding of yourself and your needs. You begin to accept the fact that you are not going to feel 100% tomorrow or next week. Try to have realistic goals for yourself. Begin to take one day at a time. Even though you probably feel very down and discouraged, try to remember that you are going to become less confused. Try to give yourself credit during this difficult time. You are working very hard.

After what seems like forever, but in fact is usually a few weeks, you will start to have some good days. This can be a difficult time because the first "bad" day after feeling somewhat better is very disappointing. Don't be surprised if you find you have been sitting on a mountain of rage once you give yourself permission to let the angry feelings out. This is really common. It can be overwhelming and scary, especially if it hits you unprepared.

If you feel very angry and see one of your children as the cause of your pain, you may see the child as bad or a "brat". When you start doing things to release your anger and begin to take breaks, this will shift and the child will no longer seem to be the problem. You may feel quite guilty about how unfairly you treated the child. It's important to remember, you were doing the best you could and you are working to change this. Even though what you were doing wasn't okay, don't be too hard on yourself.

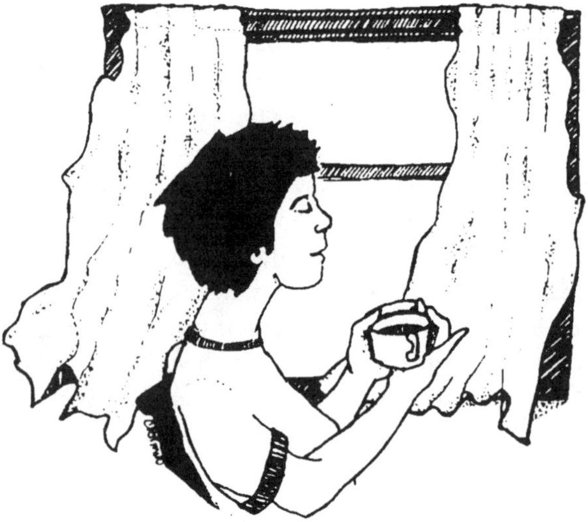

You may be aware of scary thoughts and fantasies at this time. It is possible that you are angry at your child and have fantasies in which your child gets hurt. You may be very fearful that you might hurt her or him. Try to be sympathetic with yourself; you are not a bad mother for having these thoughts and feelings. It is very important at this time to get your breaks, to express your anger safely and to talk to a trusted friend. Read and reread the chapter "What helps?" and make use of what ever ideas you can.

The scary thoughts and fantasies may be about hurting or killing yourself. Again, try to be sympathetic with yourself; you are not a bad person. Work hard at getting your breaks and dealing with your anger. Share your feelings with someone you trust. Remember, just because you have scary thoughts and feelings doesn't mean you will act upon them.

Another thing that might happen at this stage is that you become aware of some very painful memories from your past. You might have been abused as a child and now start to remember and think about that time. These memories will be very painful. Give yourself permission to cry and be angry or withdraw into yourself for a while. It's important to do whatever you feel is necessary to take care of yourself.

Fortunately, you will not only be having these scary, painful thoughts and feelings but you will also be starting to get in touch with some of your positive feelings. If you have been feeling nothing for your child, this may be the time that you have a flash of good feeling for your baby. You may find yourself smiling sometimes and perhaps regaining your sense of humour. These good feelings are usually of short duration at first. Gradually, however, they become more frequent and last for longer periods of time. It is important to make yourself take notice of these good feelings. Take time to appreciate them—you deserve to do this after all the pain you have been coping with.

Some women say, "Getting through this is like peeling an onion—going through the layers." Others describe it as a "roller-coaster ride" with some really good days followed by terrible ones. These highs and lows may seem quite extreme. When you are feeling very happy the temptation will be to assume that the depression is all over and to start making great plans. It is disappointing when the low hits and you come crashing down. This may feel like a setback, but it is quite common and part of the process. It does not undo all the work you have done so far.

Occasionally women describe themselves as being stuck—not moving backwards or forwards. When this happens all you can do is go back to basics—take your breaks, express your anger safely, nurture yourself. In time things will begin to move again.

You will gradually start to have more good days than bad. As part of keeping your expectations realistic and looking after your own needs, you will be learning how to set limits and how to say *no.* Saying *no* may be hard at first, but each time you say it you have won a victory. You will start to have more control over your life and will find that you are more able to ask for what you want and need from your partner, your friends, and others.

At this stage things start to become clearer. One woman said, "I finally began to feel as if my head was above water, as if the fog had lifted and I could see me again." You usually know what you are crying about and can start to pay more attention to doing what is right for you rather than living up to everyone else's expectations. Feeling better does not mean everything is perfect. Crises occur in all of our lives, none of us escape having "bad" days.

At this point, don't be surprised if you feel the need to explore some of the issues which may have come up during your depression. For example, if you have been sexually abused or if your parents were alcoholics, you probably have been remembering the pain of these things when you have been going through the depression. This may be the time to seek out a counsellor to deal with this unfinished business. In the chapter "Getting help from professional helpers" there are some ideas about how to select a counsellor that you can trust. If you choose to do this, keep in mind that it shows how much you have recovered: not only have you worked through a very difficult period, but you now feel strong enough to consider working through these unfinished issues.

As you get stronger you will probably realize how isolated and lonely you have felt. If you live in a small community you may have felt ashamed of your depression and may have withdrawn from community life or worn a "mask" to hide your true feelings. The realization that you have been lonely and you want this to change is an important step in getting better. Making friends with whom you can be yourself takes time and patience. Go slowly and stick with it. You deserve to have caring, supportive friends.

As you feel better you may also notice that you get some of your sexual feelings back. You will probably start to have sexual fantasies, often not about your partner. Do not be distressed by this—it is very common and simply means you are feeling sexual again; it does not mean that you are no longer attracted to your partner. Your sexual relationship will need to be rebuilt gradually, something which may take time and patience.

Many women say that they are glad they went through a postpartum depression, because they learned a lot about themselves from the experience and have grown because of it. Even though you may feel alone, it is important to remember that 10-28% of women who have a baby experience a PPD. With hard work, time and patience, you are going to get through it.

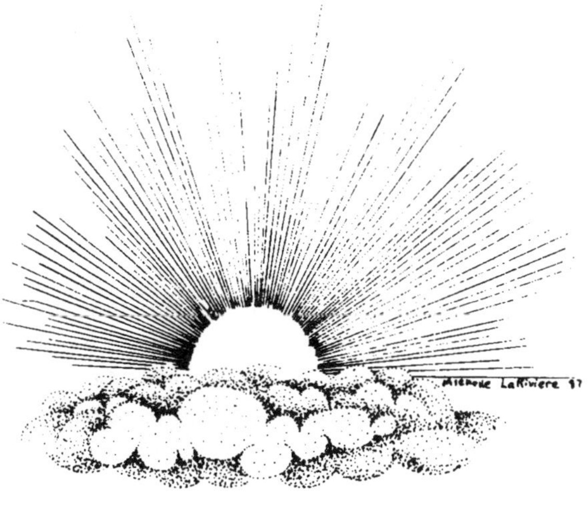

The motherhood myth

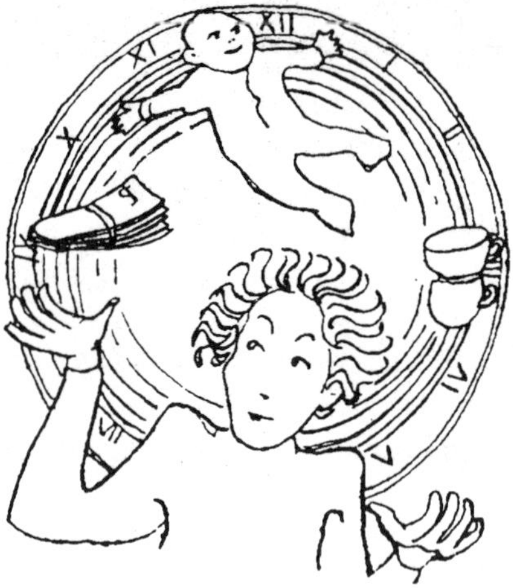

From the time they are little girls and throughout their lives, women constantly receive the message that mothers should be beautiful, serene, and radiant, as well as expert shoppers, gourmet cooks and immaculate housekeepers. "Good" mothers always have the time to play with their children and the wisdom to guide and discipline them. Furthermore, "supermom" is supposed to have infinite, constant, loving, tender and protective feelings for her baby. These feelings supposedly develop immediately after and are a consequence of giving birth, when the mother bonds with her baby. In fact, it is quite common for the bonding relationship to take place over a number of weeks or months.

In the western world, motherhood is seen as the final peak of femininity, the fulfillment of womanhood. As a result, many women who find themselves unfulfilled by mothering feel inadequate and disappointed. Those not choosing to be mothers feel forced to explain their "selfishness". Those women who are unable to have children have to cope with messages which imply that they are less than complete women.

Moreover, the mythology holds that mothering is "intuitive" and "natural". A mother is expected to respond intuitively to the baby's needs so that the baby is happy and contented and does not cry. A mother who is unsure what to do or who cannot stop her baby crying is often viewed with suspicion. She is likely to receive messages (spoken or unspoken) which imply that there is something wrong with her ability to mother.

This myth of the supermom upholds mothering as the central role for all women. Mothers are expected to place low priority on their own personal, sexual, educational and economic needs and are supposed to take care of the needs of their families first. When they look at their own experiences and compare their mothering to the image upheld by the myth, all women see themselves as failures. In trying to act the part, "to do the right thing", it is inevitable that a woman will catch sight of her harried, anxious face in the mirror. She knows she cannot measure up and assumes that she is the problem. The incredible pressure to be perfect causes many women to feel ashamed of their feelings and experiences and makes it very difficult for them to seek out and receive help. The myth of the supermom has a profound effect. It causes women to judge themselves, their mothers and their friends on its terms and makes it very difficult for women to talk to each other about the reality of their experience.

The messages women receive about mothering are very confusing. On the one hand, society glorifies and romanticizes motherhood, telling women "it is the most important job in the world". On the other hand, because mothering is supposed to be natural and intuitive, women receive no training or reward for it and get the message that there is nothing at all special about having a baby and rearing children. Women are supposedly just doing what is natural and normal. It is "as if women were born to shape healthy, happy children".[4]

The reality is that rearing children is a demanding, serious and long-term responsibility for which women are not trained. No matter what their individual experiences, most mothers agree that motherhood has profoundly changed their lives. The arrival of a child can find even an experienced mother unprepared, especially if previous births were problem-free. "Why didn't anybody tell me it would be like this?" is one of the most common questions asked in mother and child drop-in centres. As Sheila

Kitzinger says in *Women as Mothers*: "There is so little recognition of what is actually involved in the fatiguing task of being a mother that women are usually made to explain their postpartum experience entirely in terms of internal states—their hormones, their psyches and their inadequate personalities, instead of the realities of the situation, as they adjust to the new occupational and emotional tasks of motherhood—tasks that are overwhelming for every woman no matter how experienced in childcare or housekeeping and how balanced she is."[5]

Motherwork involves 24-hour-a-day responsibility, night shifts, no scheduled time off, social isolation, no job training, limited areas of decision making, monotony and absence of feedback or immediate rewards. It is a job which, like all other jobs, some enjoy and some do not. Unfortunately, unlike other jobs, those who do not enjoy it can not resign. All these factors contribute to a high stress situation. Maybe the question should not be why do some mothers get depressed, but rather how does anyone manage not to!

An important decision which has to be made by many women concerns the choice to work outside the home. Again, women receive a double message. On the one hand, society sometimes treats mothers who choose to stay at home with children as unintelligent and dull. "Everyone from the dentist to the postman treated me as if I were stupid." On the other hand, mothers who choose to do paid work are suspected of being neglectful and self-indulgent.

The financial circumstances of many women do not give them the privilege of choice. They may feel angry and resentful that they have to go out to work. Some go back before they are ready, feeling panic as to whether they can cope, but fearing the loss of their jobs if they stay away too long. Others prefer to go out to do paid work rather than being home all day. Some want to work but feel discouraged from doing so by their partners or other family members. "I would like to go back to work but my husband thinks that when you have a baby you should stay at home." Those choosing to stay home may feel very ambivalent about it. "I really want to go back to work, but I just can't leave her when she is so little. I guess I'll stay home." Other women are able to be very clear about their choice to stay at home. They can afford it and find the experience enjoyable.

What all mothers have in common is that they are dealing with an extremely complex situation. Those who stay at home often feel lonely and experience society's lack of respect; those who do paid work struggle with immense child care problems and messages that "good" mothers stay at home. The task for each woman is to sort out what is best for her. This may not be what is best for her sister or her friend, and what is best for her this year may not be so next year. Motherwork is extremely hard work, whether a woman remains at home or combines this with paid work. The myth of the supermom, who has everything she wants, is just that—a myth.

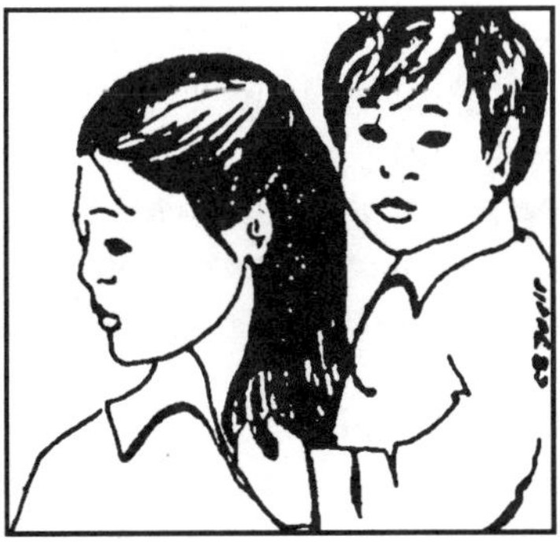

Relationships

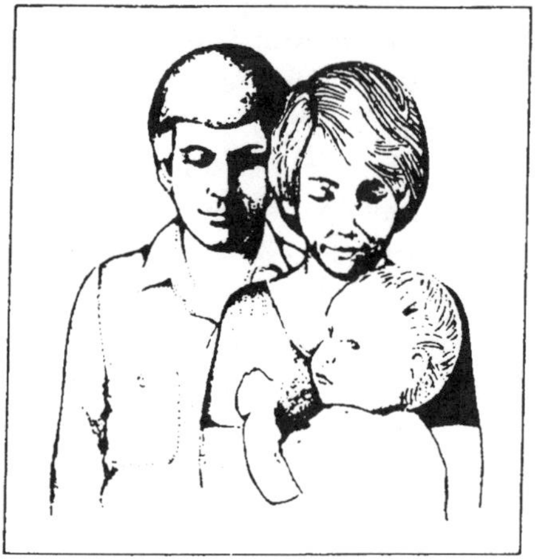

The arrival of a baby is always a time of change, transition, and possible crisis. The demands of the new baby, the broken sleep, the load of household chores, and possibly the care of older children often mean parents feel very stressed. Furthermore the emotional needs of the older children are very high at this time, placing great demands on a relationship.

In more traditional families, the father sees himself as the breadwinner; the mother, whether she is working outside her home or not, usually fulfills the traditional mother role. She does most of the housework and takes emotional responsibility for the family too. Even when couples talk before the birth about sharing the load equally, these good intentions often deteriorate when the baby is born. "I thought he'd be helpful when the baby came, but if she cries, it is always ME who deals with it."

This picture becomes more complicated if the mother feels exhausted, depressed, has low energy and is unable to deal with the baby, or if she feels anxious, and cannot slow down. Her partner often feels very confused and disappointed by the situation. He may not know what to do or say. Some men, usually those who are already doing some of the housework, try to help by doing more. The woman needs this help and feels that she should appreciate it. Often her friends tell her how lucky she is to have such a helpful husband. When he takes over more of the household tasks, however, the woman sometimes feels inadequate. Doing this work, even if it was tedious, had given her a sense of herself. The more household work he does, the more lost and like a failure she feels and she starts to resent him. At the same time the husband or partner starts to resent his mate for not coping as well as he thinks she should. A "no-win" cycle develops and puts a great strain on the relationship.

The situation can be even more complex if the man thinks that the ONLY way he can help is by doing the physical housework. He does not ask her what help she needs and wants, but instead takes control and reorganizes things his way. She is reduced to feeling childlike and powerless. It might be that what she really needs is emotional support—a hug or a listening ear. The woman may find it impossible to ask for this kind of attention. Her experience may be that any physical affection has sexual overtones, or when she asks for a hug her partner ends up being the one who is nurtured and she is left feeling drained. She may believe that her husband should know what she wants and that if she has to ask, it is not as meaningful.

Another way that a man might handle his wife's depression is by withdrawing, both emotionally and physically. He may stay at work for longer hours, go out more with his friends, or he may spend more time on his hobbies or pursuing other interests. This withdrawal leaves the woman isolated and unsupported, though at times it can be a relief from the uneasy tensions in the home when he is present. As the man leaves the house in the morning the woman may feel envious that he can escape to what seems like a comfortable job. She is left alone with the chaos, demands, and the overwhelming responsibility of the home and the children.

When a new baby is born, jealousy can arise, especially if it is the first baby. Even though, rationally, the man knows that his partner is not choosing the baby over him, emotionally he finds the loss of her undivided attention very distressing and feels in competition with the baby. Women say things like "Sometimes I feel as if I have two children, not one". This is especially difficult for the woman at those times when she feels she would like her partner to take care of her.

It can be the mother who feels jealous. It may seem to her that her partner is only interested in the baby and not in her. There seems to be a natural tendency for the other children to seek extra closeness with their father when the mother's attention is needed by the baby. This can be very painful for the woman. The toddler, with whom she has enjoyed a very close relationship, now refuses to let her help with dressing, or runs to daddy with an open show of affection while ignoring her. This is a normal process which helps the toddler to cope with the new arrival, but it can be an excruciatingly painful loss for the mother. Sometimes the mother becomes resentful of the baby because of this. "Everything was fine until the baby came. He got between myself and my daughter." It is important that the woman allow herself to grieve the loss of the special relationship which she previously enjoyed with her toddler.

When a woman is experiencing PPD it's not uncommon for her to have no sexual feelings. This can be seen by her partner as a rejection of him. At the same time, she may also be feeling unloved and think that he is only interested in her sexually and is not willing to give her the emotional support she needs. Distance may increase between them, and she may feel as if the relationship is falling apart. Some men are unable to handle the situation and may seek relationships elsewhere. Some use the threat (implied or spoken) of an affair to pressure their partners into having sex with them.

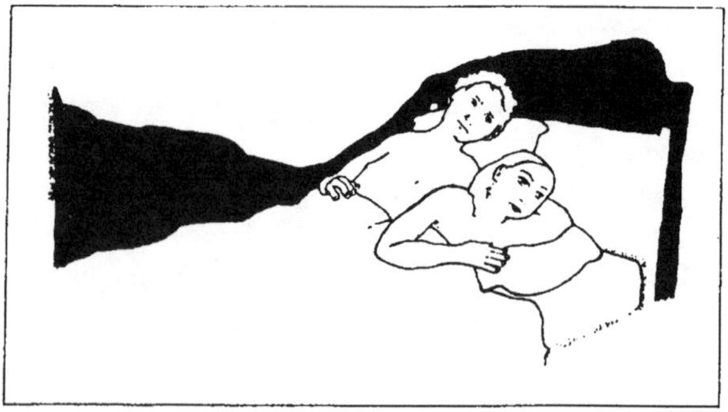

Sometimes, in his frustration and anger, the man will become verbally abusive and say such things as "You've got to snap out of it" or "It's time you pulled yourself together, you silly bitch". Some men will become physically abusive and may hit or kick the woman, or may lock her in a room, or threaten her in other ways. Most women blame themselves when this happens. A woman who is experiencing postpartum depression is especially hard on herself. She thinks she has caused the abuse because she is depressed. She usually needs a lot of encouragement and support to see that her depression does not justify her partner's abusive behaviour. If this is happening to you, call a transition house if there is one in your area and talk to a worker. You can do this even if, at this time, you do not want to go there to stay. You will find the number in the phone book. If there is no other help, at least try to phone a friend.

Even if the man is not abusive, the stresses and strains of the situation, when extended over a period of time, can cause a great deal of resentment and bitterness. This can leave the woman feeling very hopeless. As she starts to feel better, however, she often begins to be more assertive in her relationship. She is able to ask clearly for what she needs and to say *no* without being overwhelmed with guilt. Unfortunately, sometimes, as she begins to feel stronger, her partner becomes distressed about the changes he sees in her and how they will affect him. Some couples choose to seek counselling to resolve these new conflicts.

The number of women who are single parents at some time during their mothering is increasing. There is still very little written about their situation and the lower status they experience in our society. Single parents who are in contact with their former partners get varying degrees of support, ranging from financial support, to co-parenting, to nothing at all. Many find that this help and support from their ex-partner comes with a price attached—the price of sexual availability, fear of the child being kidnapped, or the threat of loss of custody. Even in a cooperative relationship, the negotiating and coordinating involved in co-parenting can take an emotional toll.

Some women wonder whether they have made the right choice by separating. The children may be acting out a lot. In addition, the isolation, insecurity and total responsibility which comes from being alone with children is very hard to cope with. Financial security is usually an issue, and the woman may look at the situation and wonder if she has made the right decision. She may be tempted to deny how unhappy she was in the relationship and may accept sexual contact, out of her need for comfort. Any woman who is considering returning to a relationship needs to ask herself if anything has really changed.

A single mother who has no active relationship with the child's father may experience guilt about having her baby. Relatives and friends may have tried to talk her out of her decision to keep the child. When the woman becomes depressed she may feel that these people were right and be uncomfortable asking for their support. Being a single parent is very difficult and, when she is feeling overwhelmed, the woman may forget or not understand that being unable to cope is part of postpartum depression. This feeling does not mean that the woman made the wrong choice when she decided to be a single parent.

When a woman is a single parent and also experiencing PPD she becomes extremely isolated. Her life becomes one long attempt to cope with all the conflicting demands upon her. It is very difficult for her to get her needs for adult relationships met. If the woman has recently left a relationship she may not be interested in starting another for a while: it takes time to work through the grief that accompanies the end of a relationship. Other women simply do not have the child care available to free up the time and energy needed to form new relationships. When a woman becomes a single parent, she usually finds that her single friends do not have the empathy or experience to give her much practical help. Generally speaking, single mothers find their best source of support from others in a similar situation.

Getting help from professional helpers

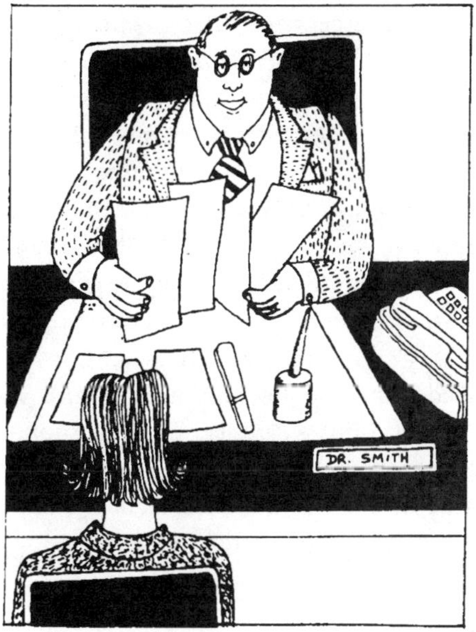

When a woman realizes that something is wrong, she may seek help from a "professional". These include public health nurses, doctors, psychiatrists, psychologists, and therapists. Women have very different experiences with different kinds of professionals, and a great deal seems to depend on the individual personalities of the people involved. Much also depends on how knowledgeable the professional is about PPD; the experience she or he has helping women through it; the professional's own biases about mothering; and her or his perceptions of the particular woman seeking help.

Many professional helpers are becoming more familiar with the issues involved with postpartum depression and are sensitive to the needs of the woman who is experiencing it. It can happen, however, that a woman may feel judged or invalidated by the professional helper to whom she turns. The woman may feel that the helper is not listening to her or that he or she simply does not understand the amount or nature of the work the woman does at home.

It is important to realize that if you don't like an individual helper or don't feel respected by her or him, it is your right to seek help elsewhere. This might be more difficult if you live in a small town where there are fewer professionals to turn to; ultimately, you may have to look for alternative sources of help. (See "Developing a support system" in the chapter "What helps?")

The first professional with whom women are likely to have contact after they return home with the baby is the public health nurse (PHN). The role of the PHN very much depends on the individual worker. Many women report that the health nurse was someone they could trust and talk to, and was someone who gave them needed information and caring advice. In rural areas especially, the health nurse can play a crucial support role for a depressed mother. Some women, however, have found it difficult to open up and talk about their feelings because the PHN seemed too busy or only interested in the baby. It is important, as with any other professional, for a woman to convey her concerns about how she is feeling.

Many women see their doctor as the appropriate professional helper in their community. Women are led to expect that doctors will know what to do about physical symptoms and will be able to relieve their anxieties, but many feel nervous about discussing their depression with the doctor. Often a woman will say, "I am fine" when asked how she is doing at the six week postpartum visit. Some women feel too ashamed or frightened to talk about the crying, the numbness or the anger; others suspect that their doctor will not be sympathetic. Frequently, women want to tell their doctor but either find it difficult to know what to say, or are "feeling better" each time they reach the doctor's office. It is generally easier for a woman to talk about physical symptoms such as backache or weight problems. Women who visit their doctor frequently, yet never directly discuss PPD, may be perceived as, and end up feeling like, hypochondriacs. It may be useful to prepare a list at home of the various things you want to discuss with the doctor. By referring to a written list, you are more likely to bring up concerns that otherwise you might forget or lose the courage to talk about.

Most doctors have little training in counselling, limited experience with women who are going through PPD, as well as limited time to focus on the real issues that lie behind the backache, insomnia or "nerves". Even with these limitations, many women have found their doctors willing to listen and be a source of support.

When women discuss their feelings directly with their doctor, some doctors are very sympathetic and reassuring, but some are not. They may dismiss the seriousness of what is being said by saying things like "It's just your hormones adjusting" or "You will feel better after a good night's sleep". This can be especially true for the woman who comes in looking well-groomed and "together". A doctor may immediately assume the woman is able to cope and just needs time to adjust. On the other hand, women who look depressed will frequently be offered medication. Some women who report having scary thoughts and fantasies find their doctors become anxious because they are unaware that fantasies are a common part of a PPD.

Many doctors that recognize the depression use medication in the form of antidepressants or tranquilizers as the first or only choice of treatment. (See the chapter "Medications—making an informed choice".) These medications are helpful for some women but confuse and complicate the picture for others. Before a woman decides whether to take medication or not, she needs to be given as much information and support as possible to help her make the right choice for herself. Whatever her choice, she will need support and understanding to get through a PPD.

Sometimes a doctor refers a mother who feels depressed or anxious to a psychiatrist, psychologist or mental health worker, who may have more experience treating PPD. However, it can be very frightening to make and keep an appointment with any of these professionals. Even though huge advances have been made in understanding the emotional needs of people, it sometimes seems that our society continues to stigmatize those who need help with emotional rather than physical problems. This can feel especially true in small towns where there is not the anonymity found in big cities.

Some psychiatrists look at a woman's past to explain her postpartum depression. They may look at the woman's childhood in order to explain her present problems—her feelings of anger or "rejection of motherhood". While there may be issues in a woman's past which come up when she is going through a PPD, this approach does not acknowledge the current stressful situation in which she is living or the social pressures on her. When a woman is in the depths of depression, it is not usually a good time for her to examine her past. She needs to feel stronger before she can do this. While depressed, the woman needs to be able to talk about what is happening now. Emphasis on her childhood can reinforce her belief that there is something wrong with her, that she is a failure as a mother and a person.

Since psychiatrists, more than other professionals, are often seen as the ultimate authority on psychological matters, they are expected to be able to tell the client what to do to recover. However, recovering from depression is a complex process and unique for each woman. No one, including a psychiatrist, has a blueprint to offer. Both the woman and society in general invest a lot of power and authority in psychiatrists—they are seen as the experts. But women have found that the healing process in postpartum depression is intimately connected with becoming "one's own expert". The woman needs to be supported to look to herself for answers and to see the choices she can make for herself.

Another of the difficulties faced by women experiencing PPD is that they are often "labelled" as being "neurotic" or having a "personality disorder". Other terms that are sometimes misused are "schizophrenic", "manic-depressive" and "psychotic". The misdiagnosis of schizophrenia is rare but has been known to occur. Occasionally a woman who is having mood swings in her depression is diagnosed as having a bipolar affective disorder (or manic-depression). Women who are having fantasies of hurting themselves or their children are at highest risk of being labelled psychotic. Having scary thoughts does NOT make a woman psychotic. Psychosis involves losing contact with reality for periods of time with no awareness of it. Psychosis usually requires hospitalization until the psychotic episode is either over or controlled by drugs. If you believe that you have been misdiagnosed, get a second opinion.

Another group of professionals or lay counsellors women turn to at this time includes pastoral workers, clergy and priests. Some women have found caring support and a strong sense of belonging through these helpers, while others have felt judged for not fitting into the prescribed maternal role and for not being able to cope.

It is important to trust your instincts. If you have a bad experience with someone, you don't need to go back. You have the right to seek someone else who is better suited to your needs. You might find the names of suitable professional helpers at a local women's health organization, or you might get recommendations from another woman that you know.

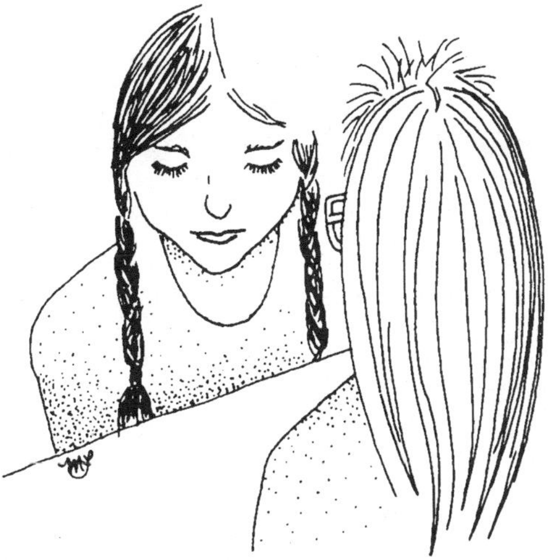

Bear in mind some basic questions when you are looking for a doctor, psychiatrist or therapist. These include:

1. Would you be more comfortable with a woman and is there one available?

2. Does this person have much personal or professional experience with postpartum depression? You can ask:
   - Do you have experience with postpartum depression?
   - Have you helped women through it? How have you helped them? (Does the doctor or psychiatrist routinely prescribe drugs?)
   - Do you relate present circumstances to the experience of postpartum depression or do you concentrate solely on the past?
3. From initial contact or first impression, is this helper able to listen to you, or is she or he denying or minimizing your feelings?
4. Does she or he speak in terms you can understand?
5. Do you feel the professional respects what you are saying?
6. Does this helper make you feel stronger or do you feel "labelled" and left confused?
7. Does this helper tell you what she or he thinks you should do, or does she help you decide what *you* think you should do?

Women who are experiencing PPD have widely varying experiences with professional helpers: sometimes they are helpful, sometimes not. You will know in a few meetings if a practitioner is right for you. If she or he is not, you can let her know that you wish to consult someone else. Keep looking—the appropriate professional helper can become a valuable member of your support system.

Medications—making an informed choice

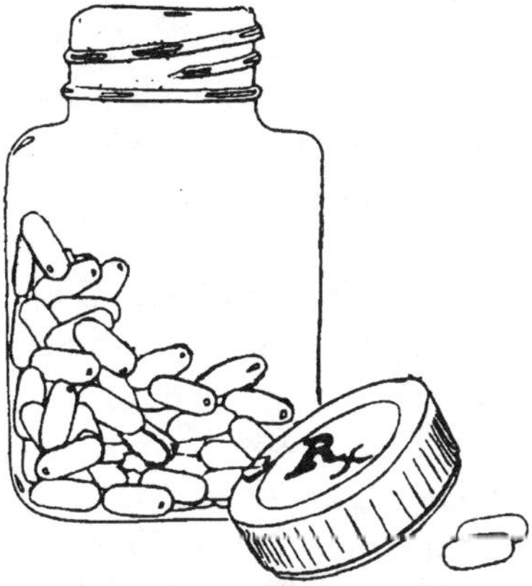

A certain amount of stress is part of daily living. Particular times in our lives are more stressful than others. In the past, people used herbs, teas and other natural remedies as a means of coping during difficult times. In this century, however, we have seen a boom in the pharmaceutical drug industry with the production of drugs such as tranquilizers and antidepressants. A large proportion of these medications are prescribed to women.

When a woman is going through a postpartum depression, these medications are often prescribed. While many women resolve their postpartum depression without the use of such drugs, others find relief from taking them. However, finding a medication which works satisfactorily is rarely simple or quick.

Each woman's body reacts slightly differently to drugs. For some women, the prescribed dosage will be helpful; for others it will have no effect. Some women experience worrying side effects from the drugs they are taking; some do not. Unfortunately, it is impossible for a woman to know what her reaction will be to a drug until she takes it. Once she is taking the medication, the woman may find it hard to distinguish what feelings are from her postpartum depression and what are side effects of the medication. Moreover, when the drug is stopped, the withdrawal symptoms can be similar to those of the anxiety and depression for which it was originally prescribed. It is very difficult to tell whether the symptoms are from the depression itself or the withdrawal from the medication.

If a woman is pregnant or breastfeeding and considering taking medication, the effects of the medication on the fetus or child must also be considered. Research on some antidepressants used during pregnancy appears reassuring so far, but more extensive and long-term studies are still needed. However, if a woman is severely depressed, and she is unable to sleep or nourish herself or is feeling suicidal, the effects of *not* taking the medication need to be weighed against any risk from the medication itself.

It is very important that a woman who is being offered or who is considering taking medication learn as much as possible about the drug so she can make an informed choice. The following information will be helpful in this regard.

Pharmaceutical drug names

A PHARMACEUTICAL DRUG has two names: the generic name (or chemical name), and the brand name given to it by the drug company which manufactures it. Medications are commonly known by their brand names. *Valium* is a brand name of the chemical diazepam. Sometimes the same drug is made by several different companies and has several brand names. For example, the anti-anxiety medication lorazepam is known by the brand names *Ativan* and *Novo-lorazem.*

If your doctor uses the generic name, your pharmacist will provide you with the cheapest form of the medication that's available. There is NO difference in the effectiveness.

Dosage

PILLS ARE USUALLY prescribed as tablets or capsules with a certain weight. The weight is commonly in milligrams (mg). One milligram is one one-thousandth of a gram. Some medications are naturally stronger than others. There is no one correct dosage. As different bodies react differently to various medications, you could easily be given a dosage which is not right for you. If the effect of the medication you are taking is distressing, ask your doctor to change the dosage. Trust your feelings and don't be afraid to question. You are the expert about your body, and you have the right to expect your doctor to take your reports seriously. It might take your doctor and you a while to arrive at the correct dosage for you.

Important things to ask your doctor

IF YOUR DOCTOR or psychiatrist prescribes medication for you, the following are some of the important questions to ask:

1. Why are you prescribing this medication for me?
2. What can I expect it to do?
3. What is its brand name and its chemical name?
4. How often and when am I to take it?
5. How long will it be before I feel any effect?
6. How will it affect the way I function at home/workplace?
7. What are the possible side effects?
8. What do I do if I miss a pill?
9. What kinds of foods or drugs interact with this?
10. How long does this medication stay in my system?
11. How long can I expect to take this medication?
12. When I stop taking this medication do I have to reduce the dosage gradually?
13. What will happen if I stop suddenly?
14. Can I expect any withdrawal problems?
15. Is the medication really necessary or are there any other alternatives?
16. What effects could this medication have on a nursing infant? Can I still breastfeed?
17. What effects could this drug have on a developing fetus? Can I take this medication if I am pregnant?

Important things to tell your doctor

WHEN YOUR DOCTOR or psychiatrist prescribes medication for you, the following are some of the important things to tell them:

1. If you have taken the medication previously and your reaction to it.
2. Any other medication you may be taking, whether by prescription or purchased over-the-counter, including herbal remedies and vitamin or mineral supplements. This is especially important if you are using amphetamines, diet pills, asthma drugs or inhalers, antihistamines, hay fever or allergy pills, pain killers, sedatives, birth control pills or street drugs.
3. If you could be pregnant.
4. If you are breastfeeding.
5. If you have a problem with alcohol.
6. If you have a heart problem or any other serious medical condition.

Things to remember for yourself

1. Make sure you have all the details written down in a way that you can easily understand so that you can refer to them later.
2. Use the dosage prescribed for you. Don't take more. Remember that if you are feeling upset or nervous, this could be a side effect of the medication. Discuss this with your doctor.
3. While your body adjusts to the medication, you may need extra practical help (eg., with minding your children).
4. Unless you have been told that it is okay, do not stop taking the medication suddenly. Always decrease the dosage gradually. Withdrawal symptoms can be very distressing.
5. Some medications can cause your periods to become irregular or to stop completely.
6. Many drugs pass through to the fetus. You need to carefully research any drug if you are pregnant.

7. Many drugs pass into the breastmilk. You need to carefully research any drug if you are nursing.
8. Your pharmacist is a good source of information. She or he usually knows in detail about a particular medication.
9. If you have a really strong reaction to a drug or if you have any of the infrequent or rare side effects, call your doctor immediately.
10. Trust yourself. You are the one who knows how your body is reacting.

Recommended resources

IT MAY NOT BE POSSIBLE to remember or write down all the information you will need in choosing—or, later, monitoring—your use of any medication. A drug reference manual (designed for non-professionals) that has been recently updated can answer many questions you might have about a particular medication. Getting the most complete information available will help you make your most informed decision.

The following guides on drugs are regularly revised. They provide information that may supplement or clarify your doctor's instructions:

Complete Drug Reference. United States Pharmacopoeia. Yonkers, N.Y.: Consumer Reports Books.

Complete Guide to Prescription and Non-prescription Drugs. H. Winter Griffith. New York: Body Press/Perigee Books.

New Guide to Prescription and Over-the-Counter Drugs. Cdn. Medical Assn. Montreal: Reader's Digest Assn. (Canada).

The PDR Family Guide to Women's Health and Prescription Drugs. Medical Economics Data (Firm). Montvale, N.J.: Medical Economics Data.

Understanding Canadian Prescription Drugs: A Consumer's Guide to Correct Use. Dorothy L. Smith. Toronto: Key Porter Books.

How the helper can help

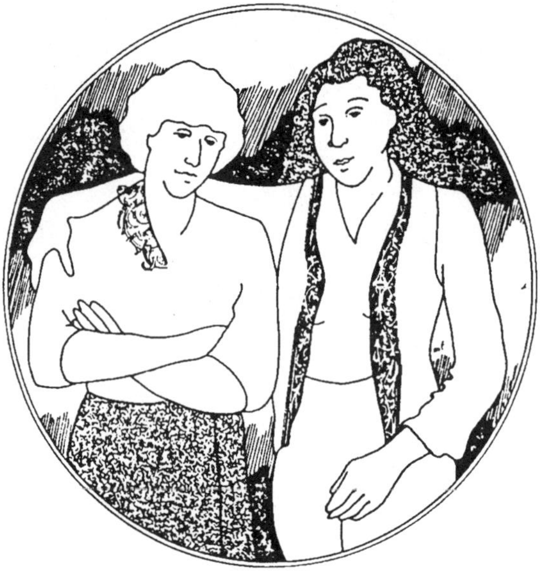

You may be reading this book because a friend or member of your family is going through a postpartum depression, or you may be a professional who is in contact with women who have young children. This chapter is intended to give you some ideas about how you can be helpful.

Practical help

THE MOTHER MAY BE asking for practical help and suggestions. The following will be useful:

- Help her to develop a simple routine for her day. Encourage her to choose one or two tasks that are manageable each day.
- Encourage her to rest whenever possible. She may not be able to sleep during the day but sitting down and having a

rest may be possible. Resting is much more important than housework.

- Encourage her to eat when she can. If she can keep a store of nutritious quick foods (cheese, cup-of-soup, fruit, yogurt) in the house, she can snack on these even if she cannot sit down to eat a meal.
- Encourage her to take breaks. Breaks are times for the mother away from the baby. Even a small break (a cup of tea when the baby is asleep) is important.
- Support her to find child care. This will be a difficult task and she may need step-by-step assistance and encouragement.
- Give her information about places she can go with her children: e.g. family places, kids' play centres, women's centres.
- Encourage her to get out of the house by herself.
- Encourage her to participate in a simple form of exercise on a regular basis, such as walking, preferably without her children.
- Invite her to go for a walk *with you.* Some people find it easier to talk about their feelings when they are walking.

Emotional support

ENCOURAGE THE WOMAN to talk to you about how she is feeling. Let her know that what she is feeling is part of the depression. She is not crazy, she is not a bad person and she is not a bad mother.

Accept her feelings

- By listening to her talk about how she is feeling, you are encouraging her to accept her own feelings. These feelings are often painful and many women want to deny them. Reassure her that accepting the feelings and allowing their expression is healing. Help her find ways of dealing with her anger safely. (See "Accepting the painful feelings" in the chapter "What helps?")

Support her decisions

- Because the woman is still learning what is right for herself and her baby, she often feels unsure about the decisions she is making. Moreover, all the information she is given can be contradictory and confusing. Give her support and encouragement about the decisions she is able to make.

Encourage her to take one day at a time

- A mother feeling depressed also feels a lot of anxiety. Consequently, she will often worry about things that have happened in the past or that may happen in the future. Help her to focus, as much as possible, on today.

Help her to redefine who she is

- Encourage her to talk about who she was before she had the baby. Ask her how this is different from who she is now. You are trying to help her identify what she has lost in order that she can grieve for this. Then she will be able to develop a renewed sense of herself.

Encourage her to give herself credit

- All women experiencing postpartum depression have high expectations of themselves and feel guilty when they do not meet them. Help her to examine her expectations and become more realistic. Remember to stress that mothering is hard work and she deserves acknowledgement for the work she does.

Share your own experiences

- If you are a mother, share your experiences with her where appropriate.

Reassure her that lack of sexual interest is normal at this time

- A lack of sexual feeling is normal in a postpartum depression. As the mother recovers, the feelings will return.

Help her to talk about this to her partner if she wants to. She needs physical expressions of affection even though she does not want to engage in sexual activity.

THE MOST IMPORTANT THING to remember when you are trying to help someone with postpartum depression is that your non-judgmental, caring support will be the most helpful. Listening to her without criticizing is much more important than saying the "right" thing or having all the answers.

When you are helping someone, remember also that you need to take care of yourself. Supporting someone who feels depressed is very hard work. Try to arrange your support for times when you will be relaxed and not likely to be interrupted. If you feel unable to provide support on a particular occasion, let the woman know that you would like to arrange another time. If you have trouble finding the time, or if you are feeling resentful or irritable with her, it is probably a sign that you are overextending yourself. You cannot help someone if you are feeling this way. It means you need to take some time to care for yourself, too.

Planning ahead

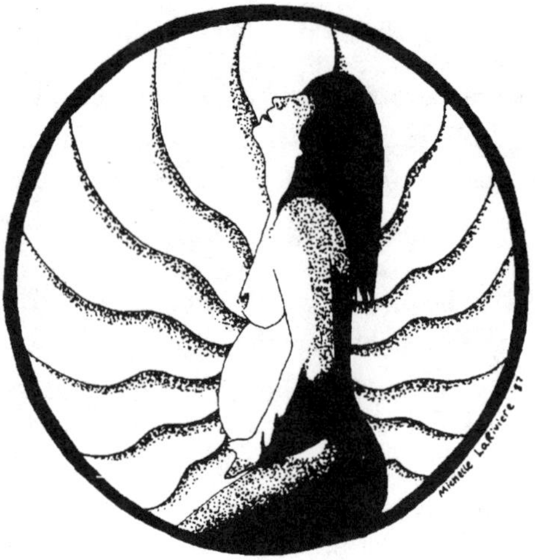

Knowing that postpartum depression can happen to one in five mothers is scary for pregnant women. In fact, depression and anxiety may start during pregnancy. When a woman has experienced one PPD she is frightened that it will happen again. Naturally everyone would like there to be a way of preventing this. Unfortunately, PPD is such a multifaceted problem that there is no one thing that you can do to prevent it. You can, however, make some preparations which may help you avoid becoming depressed and which will certainly prevent any depression from escalating.

Plan to get time for yourself

BEFORE THE BIRTH, try to make concrete plans for getting time for yourself as you may be too busy afterwards. Discuss with your partner, friends and family how they might provide you with practical help. Perhaps your mother-in-law could prepare meals for the freezer. And your sister or brother might agree to take your toddler out for a walk once a week. Do not rely on one plan for getting time to yourself. Also, do not settle for vague promises—make definite plans.

When thinking about getting time for yourself do not forget the value of small breaks. Plan to take short amounts of time when the baby is sleeping; these breaks are more important than housework. Some suggestions: Have a cup of tea, put up your feet for five minutes, step outside for a couple of deep breaths of fresh air, buy flowers for yourself at the market. (See "Nurturing yourself" and "Getting breaks" in the chapter "What helps?")

Plan to use child care

YOU WILL NEED to get time alone after you have the baby. If you have more than one child you may want, on occasion, to spend time with each of them. At these times, however, your partner may be unwilling or unable to provide child care. As well, you and he may wish to spend some time alone together. In all probability, therefore, you will need to use a child care provider.

If you can interview babysitters and other child minders prior to the birth it will make the task of getting a break much easier. Ask your public health nurse for a list of child care facilities and individuals in your community. Your public health nurse may also have a list of questions to refer to when you are interviewing prospective child care providers.

It is important to discuss with your partner that child care costs are going to be part of your budget. As a priority, child care may need to take precedence over other things.

Develop a support system

APART FROM YOUR husband or partner, who gives you support? Are any of these people in situations similar to yours (with a new baby or other children and a new baby)? Do you have someone you can really trust and with whom you can share your feelings? Have any of the mothers you know indicated that it is difficult being a mother? These are important questions to ask yourself.

You will need a support system after the baby is born. You will need women friends from whom you can seek help and advice, and with whom you can share your experiences. You might find other supportive women in prenatal classes, at women's centres, family centres, babysitting co-ops, etc. It can be very reassuring to know you have someone you can call when you are having a bad day.

It will help if you can build up such a support system before the arrival of the new baby.

Examine your beliefs and expectations

ASK YOURSELF HOW YOU would describe a "good" mother. You will probably find yourself answering with sentences such as "a good mother should always be patient"; "a good mother should always be gentle with her child"; "a good mother should always provide nutritious meals".

When you have identified your beliefs, ask yourself where they come from. Where did you learn that a good mother should always be patient? From books? From the fact that your own mother was often impatient with you and this upset you? You will get a good deal of information about yourself by examining your beliefs about mothers.

The next step after examining these beliefs is to sort them out. You may believe that patience is a virtue in mothers and unrealistically expect yourself to be patient all the time. It may help you to identify what circumstances make it easy for you to be patient. What circumstances make it difficult? If you are more likely to be impatient when you are rushed, it will be important for you to try to pace yourself as much as you can. However, as a mother you will sometimes be rushed and therefore impatient.

Finally, try to restate your expectations of yourself in more realistic terms. Remember: just as your baby will grow and develop, so will your mothering and parenting skills. Becoming aware of your beliefs about mothering and more realistic about what you can expect of yourself will help you avoid judging yourself harshly and reduce the stress that this entails.

Wait before you decide whether you will return to your job

WHEN YOU ARE PREGNANT you may feel sure that you do not want to return to your job. Alternatively, you may feel sure that you do. If possible, do not make any final decisions until a few months after the birth. Many women are surprised at how their feelings about working can change after the birth of their child. Give yourself as much time as you can to make the decision. It is an important one, and needs to be right for *you.*

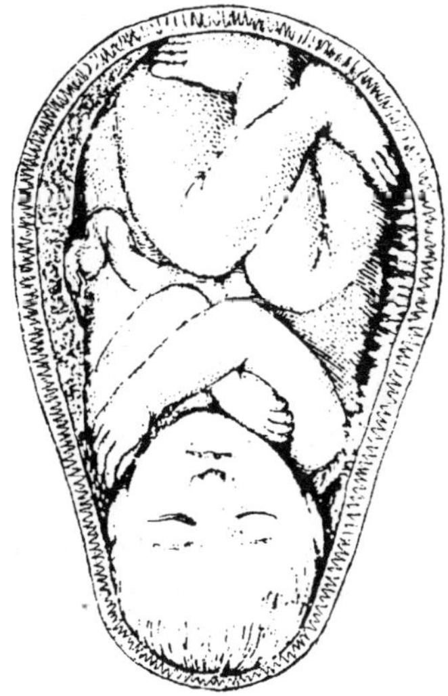

Be flexible with your birth plans

WHEN PLANNING YOUR birth experience, inform yourself as much as possible about your options. The more informed you are, the more choice and control you will have over the birth. Read, go to childbirth classes, talk to other mothers, do anything you can to inform yourself and to develop your own birth plan. If you can, create your own birth plan, in writing, and give it to the hospital when you register.

When you have done your preparation you have done all you can do. You can never predict with total accuracy how a birth will go. All you can do, once the birth starts, is to stick to the birth plan where you can and let go of the parts which aren't working; take care of yourself as much as possible; do the best you can and hope that everything will go smoothly. You cannot control the whole process.

You may be fortunate and have a satisfying birth experience. You may be unfortunate and run into medical complications or disrespectful medical staff. You are not to blame if things do not go as planned. Remember this when you are thinking about your birth experience. If things do not go as you had hoped, remaining as flexible as possible will help you cope.

Take your own needs into account when making decisions about the postpartum period

WHEN YOU ARE MAKING decisions about issues such as breastfeeding, it is important to think not only about the baby but also about yourself. You may believe that breastfeeding is best for the baby. You may also feel very trapped by the constant demands this will make on you. If this is the case, think about compromises such as primarily breastfeeding and, when your milk is established, giving one bottle a day, or one or two bottles a week. This will enable someone else (your partner or friend) to feed the baby, and give you a chance to take care of yourself (sleep, have a relaxed bath, go out alone for a few hours). If you or the father have allergies, consult your doctor or allergist before introducing any kind of supplement.

You may find yourself in similar conflict if you have the choice of the baby rooming in or not. You may feel that rooming in will help you to bond with your baby, while at the same time you know you will have little opportunity to rest when you return home. Again think about a compromise. Maybe you can have rooming in and send the baby to the nursery when you want to sleep or bathe.

The main thing to remember when facing these types of problems is that YOUR NEEDS ARE IMPORTANT. Do not base your decisions solely on the needs of the baby.

Evaluate your previous postpartum experiences

IF YOU HAVE EXPERIENCED a postpartum depression after a previous birth it may be frightening to think of risking another birth. Considering the pain endured, these feelings are very real and understandable. While a depression can occur after any birth, a woman who has resolved a previous depression will have a better understanding of what is happening to her should she experience one again. As well, she will have acquired skills that will help her through another difficult postpartum adjustment.

If you still have a lot of painful feelings and memories left from your previous experience, it may be a good idea to look for some counselling to help you sort them out. Do not be afraid or ashamed to ask for this help. You will be able to cope much better with successive births.

If you have previously experienced a postpartum depression and have worked through it, you will have learned a lot. You probably know more about yourself and about ways of taking care of yourself (nurturing yourself, getting breaks, accepting your feelings). If you have developed these skills, they will prove very useful to you.

Consider the possibility of PPD

SPEND SOME TIME discussing with your partner that PPD and anxiety is a possibility. Even if you do everything you can to prevent it, there is always the possibility that it will occur. PPD is such a multidimensional problem that it is not possible to think about and prepare for every eventuality.

It will help if you spend some time planning what you will do if you get depressed and/or anxious. Will your partner be able to stay at home with you for a while? Can you ask someone to stay with you to help you? Do you have a doctor or other helper who is knowledgeable in this area and who will treat you appropriately if you do experience postpartum depression? The more planning you do, the more equipped you will be to handle the situation.

Women's stories of recovery

Every woman's story of recovery from postpartum depression is unique. The point at which a woman realizes "things are not quite right", what motivates her to seek help, and the steps she takes in the process of recovery, all vary from woman to woman.

The four women whose stories follow found support from a variety of sources to help them resolve their postpartum depression and anxiety.

Maureen

MY FIRST CHILD, MY DAUGHTER, *recently turned twelve years old. It amazes me to realize that ten years have passed since I first sought help for the extreme distress I had been battling for close to two years.*

My unexpected difficulties began in the hospital. After my perfect pregnancy, an ideal labour and the easy birth of my beautiful baby girl, I thought the hard part was over. However, sleep eluded me, breastfeeding was painful and there weren't enough hours in the day to care for my newborn and myself. My tears started when the first visiting hour came and went without a visitor—everyone wanted to let me rest! I thought this was just the "baby blues" and expected to regain control in a few days. But once we got home, my daughter developed colic, and was constantly uncomfortable, sleepless and miserable. Nothing comforted her and I began to feel totally inadequate.

I remember my need to appear to be coping well. No one knew the extent of my suffering. I would sit and nurse my baby all day and watch the mess pile up around me. I felt depressed and immobilized by the growing chaos. I could not find the time to meet my most basic needs—to eat or to have a quick shower. I was overwhelmed almost all of the time. Occasionally, I was able to "get it together" and managed to shower, dress and feed myself and my daughter, but then I raced around, anxiously trying to make up for what I felt was lost time. I was always tense and couldn't relax no matter how hard I tried. I expected things to settle down after the first three months (everyone said they were the hardest), but when there was no obvious change at that time, I gave up hope. I started to feel angry and to have terrible fantasies of hurting myself or my baby. I hated myself for my inadequacies and my angry behaviour.

My husband became more and more baffled in the months after our daughter's birth. His sexual advances were furiously turned down. He felt so rejected. Our relationship really began to suffer as did my relationships with friends and family. I felt as though no one could understand me.

I tried desperately to get my doctor to "see" and "hear" me during my baby's many follow-up appointments. I constantly complained to him about how I felt. I was so run down and exhausted that I seemed to catch every virus going around. He only asked how we were managing financially since I was not working. He had no idea what I was suffering from or how to support me.

For two years I denied to myself that I could be experiencing postpartum depression. I knew it existed as I had supported a close friend through it, years before having a child of my own. My experience was so different to hers that I never related it to what I was feeling.

My anger exploded one night and I lashed out (verbally) at a close family member. I lost control and that is when I knew I needed help. I called the postpartum support organization that my friend had told me about. Talking to someone there helped me realize I wasn't alone—or crazy. I felt heard, understood and validated for the first time since the birth of my baby. There was a waiting list for their support groups—but I needed help immediately! They referred me to a therapist who specialized in postpartum issues. Thankfully, she turned out to be just right for me.

My therapist encouraged me to take a nurturing break every day—to go for a walk by myself, looking at the trees around me while breathing deeply. As basic as this sounds, it was incredibly difficult for me to do. Eventually, I began to enjoy it and little by little it became easier.

My weekly therapy session was my lifeline. I talked, cried, did "angerwork" (screamed, hit a pillow, wrung a towel) and was nurtured by my therapist. We discovered that childhood issues had actually resurfaced during my pregnancy and along with them, my rage. The angerwork helped me to focus my anger where it belonged, not at my daughter.

When a space came up in a support group, I wasn't sure I needed it anymore. My therapist encouraged me to go—to be with other mothers who were experiencing feelings similar to mine. It was scary at first but sharing with other women turned out to be a great gift. It was a relief to share my deepest thoughts and feelings with my peers and not be judged.

As I recovered, I started seeing my daughter for the delight she was rather than the focus of my pain. Our relationship improved and we had fewer power struggles. I really began to enjoy her. My husband and I took a parenting course together after I left my support group. We got a babysitter for the first time since becoming parents and went out for coffee afterwards. The first steps to getting our marriage back on track proved fruitful. A year later we were ready to expand our family.

I was nervous about having another child even though we felt ready. I worried about having another postpartum depression. Reassured by the knowledge I had gained through my PPD and by having a support network and self-care plan in place, we decided to go ahead. I am so grateful we took the risk. Our son added a sense of balance to our family. I did not experience another PPD; in fact I was able to enjoy his infancy.

While I was pregnant, my husband and I had planned how we could maximize my rest during the early postpartum period. I had already learned that rooming-in was not the healthiest choice for me, so Jim slept downstairs with our baby near him. When our son awakened for a feeding, Jim brought him to me (blissfully asleep!) then he went back to his bed. I fed our baby while lying down, both of us very relaxed and still half asleep. I only changed his diaper at night when absolutely necessary. Then it was my job to settle him in his bed downstairs. If he did not settle quickly, I called on his father for help and went back to bed! This method worked very well for all of us. I was able to sleep beautifully, not having to be on alert for my baby's cry. I also felt supported by Jim because he actively shared in the responsibility of caring for our newborn. This was very different from the first time when I felt obliged to provide all the care for our infant.

I have had other personal setbacks over the years, but none as debilitating as my PPD. *Stress has a way of creeping back into my life as I struggle to find the balance between doing too much and doing too little. I continue to learn what my limits are and to experiment with setting boundaries around what I will give and what I will take. Unfortunately, the scales tipped again while caring for my mother and having to face her terrible illness. I was also caring full time for my two young children and that meant there was nothing left over for me. I got lost in depression again. This time, the knowledge and skills I had gained through resolving my* PPD, *as well as the love and support I received from my network of friends and family, helped me to recover quickly.*

I am able to read my own warning signs of stress quite well now and, through using the self-care skills I have learned, I am able to get what I need to maintain my balance. Usually it means cutting down on my commitments and getting back to my basic needs—nurturing breaks, rest, exercise, good nutrition and talking it out with someone I trust—the first things to go when I am too busy or feeling overwhelmed. I also allow myself lots of recovery time after a particularly busy or stressful period in my life, before picking up the pace again.

I have wondered from time to time what effect, if any, my PPD *may have had on my daughter. When I look back on the videos of her first two years of life and see how sweet she was, I ask myself,* Where was I? *I was detached somehow. Whether this had any lasting effect will always be a mystery. But if I catch myself worrying about this when I see my daughter occasionally struggle with issues, I check in with friends to see if their children have similar problems. I've learned over the years that her struggles are a normal part of any child's development. At age twelve, my daughter is thriving. My improved self-esteem and the communication and self-care skills I gained while resolving my* PPD *have had, I believe, a far greater effect on her.*

When I talk about my postpartum depression, my daughter sometimes asks if she was the cause. I reassure her that she definitely was not. She was the only joyous thing about my life at that time! I believe the main causes of my PPD *were sleep deprivation, having extremely high expectations of myself, and my outrage at unresolved, painful childhood issues.*

Reflecting back over the years, I realize I am grateful for my postpartum depression. Without it, I may never have learned to care for myself or to relate well to others. I have found renewed faith in myself and great purpose in my life. My growth has enabled me to set and achieve new goals. My husband and I have recently realized our long-time dream of building our own home from where I write my story. Ten years ago, nothing could have convinced me that any of this was possible.

Alison

ALISON'S DAUGHTER WAS born six years ago after a difficult labour and delivery.

Things were difficult almost right from the beginning. I was denied medication throughout my labour. I felt like I didn't have any control over what was happening and I was being told how and when I would have my baby. I suffered a fourth-degree extension (a severe vaginal tear) during the delivery, and only then was I given a morphine IV while they were stitching me up.

I spent my first Mother's Day in the hospital. By that evening, I was in tears because I couldn't cope with trying to breastfeed and with feeling pressured to bathe, feed and change my daughter on schedule. After an unsuccessful episode with an electric breast pump, and fearing there wasn't enough time to bathe my daughter before she went to sleep, I was reassured by a kind nurse that tomorrow would still come if my baby wasn't bathed that night. She told me that I just had the "baby blues".

Things got worse when I got home. I had a very wakeful baby who was quite unhappy when she was awake. I got very little sleep and as a result, every time I was awakened during the night, I would get extremely angry and yell at my husband. I would put more pressure on myself that I wasn't doing a good job. I felt extremely inadequate and self-conscious of myself as a Mum. I felt totally disorganized, the house was a mess, breastfeeding wasn't as easy as everyone said it was, and the baby wouldn't take a bottle from my husband.

I felt trapped. I found it extremely difficult to get out of the house. I felt isolated. I thought I was the worst mother in the whole world and I felt sorry for my daughter, that she had me for a mother. I felt she was being cheated out of a good Mum and therefore would have a lousy life. I come from a dysfunctional family and have lived with the results of that. It was extremely important for me to be a perfect parent, and provide the perfect family. In my eyes, I was a failure.

I had anger and sadness at the loss of my perfect idyllic home life with my baby. Nothing was the way I expected it would be. I had no immediate bonding with my baby. I remember distinctly not liking her very much in the middle of the night. That also made me feel guilty. I didn't think that anyone else felt that way.

I was filled with "shoulds". I never trusted my instincts. I thought everyone else knew what was best for my baby. I would trust anyone's opinion except my own. The public health nurse made me feel like I was a bad Mum too. I couldn't get the baby to nurse for any more than five minutes a side, ever! I was told that meant she wasn't getting the hindmilk and her brain wouldn't develop. More guilt!

I saved most of my anger for my husband. I guess that was because I knew I couldn't take it out on my daughter. He put up with a lot. I would call him at work telling him how depressed I was, how tired I was, how badly I wanted him to be home. I watched the clock until he walked in the door. If he was a minute late, I was furious. My husband had a hard time understanding why I wasn't happy. We had planned for a long time to have this baby. We wanted this baby more than anything. I didn't understand it either. I felt helpless. I felt gross, overweight, ugly and exhausted.

When my daughter was four months old, I was feeling consumed by the anger and the sleep deprivation. I finally broke down in my doctor's office and asked for help. She recommended counselling and gave me the number for PPPSS. My first phone call to the Society was an eye-opener: I am NOT *a bad Mum; it* IS *a tough job; I* DO *deserve to get more sleep; I am* NOT *crazy; and I am* NOT *alone. I cried all through that phone call and for a long time after. It was an enormous relief. I talked about my fears about screwing up my daughter's future, and was told that by reaching out for help, I* WAS *being a good Mum.*

I used the support group to cry and talk about my feelings of anger, sadness and anxiety. It was the only place I could talk about these things because I was afraid to tell anyone else that I was depressed. I thought they would think I was weird or, worse, that I didn't love my child.

Things slowly got better, but not without a lot of hard work. I started to identify patterns, such as when my back was sore, I would get angry and yell at my husband; and that my anxiety increased before a visit from the in-laws.

I started to do angerwork to safely release my built-up anger. I started asking for my needs to be met. I learned to take breaks, which not only helped me, but also helped me to be a better mother and wife. I learned to say no *when I felt* no.

My daughter is now six years old (with a VERY *well developed brain) and I am enjoying her tremendously. I realize now that bonding for me was not an instantaneous event, but continues to build every day. People say to me, "You're so lucky, she's so well adjusted." It wasn't luck at all: it was a constant difficult job.*

I am pleased to add that my marriage is still intact and improving all the time.

Linda

TEN YEARS AGO I ATTENDED *a postpartum support group, after the birth of my third son. Looking back, I realize that I had also experienced PPD after the birth of my first son.*

In the year following the birth of my first son I felt vulnerable, irritable and overwhelmed. As time passed, I felt lonely, lacking in direction. I became panicky and worried, looking ahead into the future. What if my depression ruined my child's life, or my marriage? What if I never got any better? Would I always feel like this? I became sleepless, waking in the early hours feeling frightened and agitated. I had vague thoughts of suicide—no plans, just a deep need for peace. I had no appetite. I lost weight. I had a constant sense of doom. I was in a state of constant anxiety. I had panic attacks. I became somewhat agoraphobic and I was fearful of certain activities, such as going to the dentist, eating in a restaurant, being a passenger in a car, travelling away from home.

I saw my doctor, who was not knowledgeable about postpartum adjustment difficulties; I attended a day program at the hospital; I saw a psychiatrist. No one suggested that what I was experiencing was postpartum depression and anxiety. After several more months my doctor prescribed antidepressants and I started attending a panic disorder group. The medication helped in lowering the anxiety and fear. I began to sleep better. This helped end the cycle of anxiety, sleeplessness, fearful thinking and depression. I slowly began to heal.

I have some difficult memories of being short-tempered with my child when I was depressed. I was so sleep deprived and exhausted that I was often irritable. It didn't happen often but I have memories, which still make me regretful and sad, of being too harsh with such a tiny human being.

When my son was five years old, I became pregnant with our second son. I was still shaky but doing better. During my pregnancy I worried: Am I recovered enough to manage another child?

After our second child was born, I took time away from work and enjoyed my two sons. I did have some anxiety in the first few days after delivery but thankfully this passed quickly. It seemed that I once again had some balance in my life and I enjoyed motherhood.

A year later I became pregnant a third time. I was excited and told myself, It will be fine, I've done this before. *But at times during my pregnancy I felt depressed and anxious. I was afraid of the added responsibilities that caring for a new baby would bring, and saddened that I would have less time to spend with my other boys. I would be so busy—my two youngest would be less than two years apart. At the same time, I grieved over not being able to return to work: child care for three children would be too costly. I felt a sense of being trapped.*

Shortly after the birth of my third son, I began to feel symptoms of anxiety and depression. He was born a month early. At first he seemed content, but at two weeks old he started to cry and it seemed he didn't stop for two years. He was very colicky, difficult to breastfeed, and sensitive to many formulas. I was up day and night; he cried, I cried. Again I began to feel submerged in the feelings I had experienced before. I worried incessantly about my newborn. I awoke with frightful thoughts about the things that could happen to my children and to me. I awoke with that familiar feeling of doom.

During my second bout with PPD, I again became short-tempered with my older children—they seemed so big, didn't they know I needed them to behave perfectly?! My marriage became a mess. We resented each other for not doing enough, for not coping, for not knowing what to do.

I had received a Pacific Post Partum Support Society pamphlet from the hospital and when my third son was three months old, I contacted PPPSS and was wait-listed for a support group. I talked with someone who gave me credit for all the things I was doing taking care of my children; who didn't tell me to smarten up; who didn't tell me to try harder; and who didn't tell me how lucky I was. I felt a sense of relief and safety from that very first contact. Everywhere else I tried to talk about this I was met with the attitude that I was complaining ... that this is what mothers did ... that other mothers had done it so why couldn't I? I felt like a failure.

After I joined the PPPSS support group, things began to change and gradually improve. I sat in a room with other women who were perplexed by what was going on for them. I began to unravel the tangled threads of my postpartum adjustment experiences. I learned that it wasn't my kids' fault and that it wasn't mine or my husband's either; I began to see my husband and children more clearly as the precious beings they are; my husband and I began to rebuild our relationship. I also became aware of the reality that motherwork is challenging work. Attending the group started me on a profound road to recovery and understanding.

When my son turned one, I left the group. My life was still challenging but I now had some new ways of coping with it all. I felt a sense of healthy control. I had learned some valuable skills. I had difficult days after that, but never the desolation I had once known. I began to value myself, form supportive relationships and take care of myself—resting when the children napped, taking a relaxing bath with a lit candle. When things got rough I would go out on my front step and take deep breaths of fresh air. And I gave myself a pat on the back often. I learned that the myths of motherhood can get you in big trouble (myths like "good mothers never get angry"; "women instinctively know how to be mothers"; "I should be able to anticipate my children's needs"). As a mom, I had to write my own description of motherhood and not buy into common motherhood myths. As my children have grown and developed, I have written and rewritten my "job description" many times. Just as childhood is developmental, so is mothering.

When people ask me why I had postpartum depression, I tell them that there were many contributing factors: lack of knowledge and support; my high expectations of myself; sleep deprivation (none of my children slept through the night until they were at least one year old); hormonal changes; myths; isolation; loneliness; lack of parenting skills; secrecy; past issues; marital stress; and lack of family involvement.

It may sound strange but I have felt grateful for my experience. I have continued on in support work and education regarding postpartum issues. During that time and since, I have met so many inspiring, beautiful and courageous women. It was a long road to recovery and I'm proud of how far I've come and of the many skills I've gained turning this whole thing around.

Sharon

SHARON EXPERIENCED postpartum depression almost seven years ago after the birth of her first child.

My early postpartum experience might best be described as subsisting. *My daily goals included staying awake enough to feed and change my baby. Sleep deprivation became my number one enemy. I walked around hunched over like a ninety year old woman. With little to no sleep I was shaky, weak, headachy, paranoid, irritable, teary, unmotivated and I suffered blackouts upon rising too quickly.*

In between my child's frequent cries for food, changing and holding, I waited on pins and needles—knowing it would not be long until his next cry. Many calls to my husband at work, begging him to come home early, or "right this minute", increased my self-loathing at being so helpless.

Even when my child started sleeping through the night, my internal clock would not allow me to sleep, being trained to breastfeed every hour and a half by my infant's needy cries.

I bottomed out, wanting to just disappear with vague suicidal plans to just drive my car into a brick wall. I mistakenly believed everyone would be better off without me. I was desperate.

Throughout this period, well-meaning family members would drop in to "help", expecting tea and side-stepping the colossal mess that once was an orderly house. They suggested getting up and exercising. I felt angry at their suggestions. What I really needed was help with cleaning and child care while I slept. However, I didn't know how to ask for help yet, and they didn't know how to offer it.

Somehow I kept going. It wasn't until the birth of my second child that I finally broke the silence about my postpartum depression with a good friend, who then confided that she too had suffered a mild PPD. She gave me the phone number of a postpartum support organization.

I was scared to call, but I was glad I did. I cried and cried on that first phone call and not once was I told to "pull my socks up" or "get a hold of myself" or "just go to bed if you're sick". Instead I received reassurance—I was not going crazy, I deserved support, it was not my fault, and best of all, that things would get better.

When I was able, I joined a support group and found women just like myself who felt validated and supported by the other women's stories. A telephone support volunteer connected with me once or twice a week and soon my suicidal feelings diminished and disappeared. I discovered what I needed in my recovery process and how to get it. I hired babysitters. I hired house cleaners. At one point I hired a college student as a "mother's helper", because what I needed landed somewhere between babysitter and housekeeper and friend. I asked my husband and my friends for more help with chores and child care. Sometimes I hated needing so much help. I was constantly adjusting and fiddling with the balance between what I was needing and how much help I could tolerate. Hiring help brought its own set of problems such as setting hours and salary, and dealing with personalities and explanations of schedules and chores. It was worth the effort in the end.

I took a three week trip to my sister's house alone. Although I knew I needed to go, leaving my babies with my husband and babysitters was a big decision. While I was away I slept like a baby, pampered myself, and got up late every day. I took long baths and dressed slowly. I took vitamins and ate nourishing food. My sister and I talked when she got home from work each day and we went for walks together. I read lots of books on nutrition and would often go to bed at a very early hour. I started to feel renewed and slowly my strength returned. It was then that I started to miss my family and knew I was ready to go home.

When I got back I returned to the support group, and I began discovering other ways to nurture myself. This involved discovering and rediscovering my many passions. Reading, writing, swimming, socializing, and many other interests opened up to me once again. I recognized what my "good mother" myths were and where I could lower my expectations of myself and others. I also recognized how not to take on others' expectations of me, with as little guilt as possible.

Experiences from when I was growing up resurfaced and I sought out one-on-one help from a counsellor to deal with it. My partner and I received marriage counselling because our marriage had been under tremendous strain for too long and the threads of communication were tenuous at best.

The postpartum support organization provided support and information for my partner, and ongoing telephone support for me. Their support empowered me: I felt like the decisions leading to my new found health came from me and a real understanding of my unique needs.

Things have really changed for me now. I enjoy my children so much and have worked hard to maintain a balance between their needs and mine. I have learned that giving to myself is not selfish. When I nurture myself, I also nurture my family. If I find myself feeling blue or angry and oppressed now, I usually find I've had very little time to myself. I treat these feelings as red flags – warnings – and put my feet up, grab a nice cup of tea, and have a hard look at what I need to get back on track.

IN THE LAST FEW YEARS, women who have gone through a postpartum depression have begun to talk more about their experiences. At the same time, health care practitioners have greatly increased their understanding and recognition of postpartum depression and anxiety. The general public, as well, has become more aware of PPD. This means that now you can find knowledgeable support in many more places.

If you would like to tell us what helped you get through a postpartum depression, or if you have feedback about *A self-help guide for mothers*, we would like to hear from you. Our address is at the end of this guide.

Resources

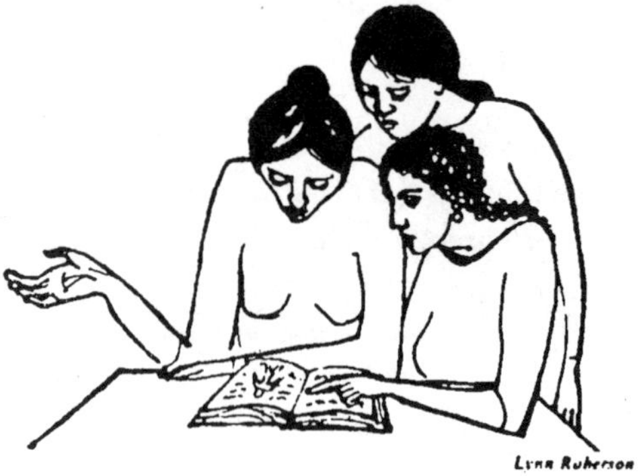

Books you might find useful

BARETT, N. (1997). *I wish someone had told me: A realistic guide to early motherhood.* Chicago: Academy Chigago Publishers.

BLOCK, J. (1991). *Motherhood as metamorphosis: Change and continuity in the life of a new mother.* New York: Plume.

THE BOSTON WOMEN'S HEALTH BOOK COLLECTIVE. (1992). *The New our bodies, ourselves.* New York: Simon & Schuster.

BROWN, S., [ET AL]. (1994). *Missing voices: The experience of motherhood.* Melbourne; New York: Oxford University Press.

DIX, C. (1988). *The new mother syndrome: Coping with post-partum stress and depression.* New York: Pocket Books.

DUNNEWOLD, A. & SANFORD, D.G. (1994). *Postpartum survival guide.* Oakland: New Harbinger Publications.

EISENBERG, A., MURKOFF, H., & HATHAWAY, S. (1989). *What to expect the first year.* New York: Workman Publishing.

___. **(1991).** *What to expect when you're expecting.* New York: Workman Publishing.

HAMILTON, J.A. & HARBERGER, P.N., (EDS.). (1992). *Postpartum psychiatric illness: A picture puzzle.* Philadelphia: University of Pennsylvania Press.

HOFFMAN, J., [ET AL]. *Hands on dad: A guide for new fathers.* Booklet in *Parenting for Life* series. Toronto: Today's Parent Group.

JACKSON, M. (1992). *The mother zone: Love, sex and laundry in the modern family.* New York: H. Holt and Co.

KENDALL-TACKETT, K. (1993). *Postpartum depression: A comprehensive approach for nurses.* Newbury Park, CA: Sage Publications.

KITZINGER, S. (1980) *Women as mothers.* New York: Vintage Books.

___. **(1994).** *The year after childbirth: Surviving and enjoying the first year of motherhood.* Toronto: HarperCollins.

___. **(1995).** *Ourselves as mothers: The universal experience of motherhood.* Reading, Mass.: Addison-Wesley.

KLEIMAN, K.R. & RASKIN, V.C. (1994). *This isn't what I expected: Recognizing and recovering from depression and anxiety after childbirth.* New York: Bantam Books.

LOUDEN, J. (1995). *The pregnant woman's comfort book : A self-nurturing guide to your emotional well-being during pregnancy and early childhood.* San Francisco: HarperSanFrancisco.

___. **(1992).** *The woman's comfort book : A self-nurturing guide for restoring balance in your life.* San Francisco: HarperSanFrancisco.

MATTHEWS, A.M. (1995). *Excited, exhausted, expecting: The emotional life of mothers-to-be.* New York: Berkeley Pub. Group.

MISRI, S. (1995). *Shouldn't I be happy: Emotional problems of pregnant and postpartum women.* New York: The Free Press.

OAKLEY, A. (1980). *Becoming a mother.* New York: Schocken Books.

O'HARA, M. (1995). *Postpartum depression: Causes and consequences.* New York: Springer-Verlag.

PACIFIC POST PARTUM SUPPORT SOCIETY. (1997: 4TH ED.). *Postpartum depression and anxiety: A self-help guide for mothers.* Vancouver: Pacific Post Partum Support Society.

___. **(1997).** *Angoisse et dépression post-partum : Un guide pratique pour les mères.* (French language translation of 3rd edition of *Post Partum Depression and Anxiety*). Vancouver: Pacific Post Partum Support Society.

___. **(1997).** *Self-help groups for women with post partum depression and anxiety: A group facilitator's manual.* Vancouver: Pacific Post Partum Support Society.

PLACKSIN, S. (1997). *Mothering the new mother: Women's feelings and needs after childbirth: A support and resource guide.* New York: Newmarket Press.

PRICE, J. (1988). *Motherhood: What it does to your mind.* London: Pandora.

RICH, A. (1976 repr. 1986). *Of woman born: Motherhood as experience and institution.* New York: Norton.

ROSSITER, A. (1989). *From private to public: A feminist exploration of early mothering.* Toronto: Inland Womensource.

SAPSTED, A.M. (1991). *Banish post-baby blues: All the advice, support and encouragement you need to cope with post-natal depression.* Great Britain: Thorsons Publishing Group.

SCHWARTZ, J.D. (1993). *The mother puzzle: A new generation reckons with motherhood.* New York: Simon and Schuster.

SWIGART, J. (1991). *The myth of the bad mother: The emotional realities of mothering.* New York: Doubleday.

TAYLOR, V. (1996) *Rock-a-by baby: Feminism, self help, and postpartum depression.* New York: Routledge.

THURER, S. (1994). *The myths of motherhood: How culture reinvents the good mother.* Boston: Houghton Mifflin.

Videos

FOR INFORMATION ON the most current videos available on postpartum depression and anxiety and on related topics, contact the organizations listed in the section "Postpartum support organizations".

Other useful resources

TO GET MORE INFORMATION on the resources available in your community, the following suggestions may be useful:

- Ask your family doctor and people working at your local health unit.
- You can find the telephone numbers of various services/organizations such as transition houses, women's shelters, crisis lines, women's organizations, family resource centres and social services by consulting your local phone book (often in the Yellow Pages) or a community resources directory available through your local library. Specific listings may be found under such section headings as *Crisis Centres, Social Service Organizations,* or *Women's Organizations.* Check the index at the back of the directory for page directions to a particular section.
- In some communities, you can call an Information Services telephone number for information on the services available from agencies in your area.
- Talk to other mothers.

Transition houses

TRANSITION HOUSES PROVIDE temporary shelter for women and their children who are in danger from physical or emotional domestic violence. They also offer individual and group counselling, telephone support, referrals and information, as well as other services related to family violence or mental cruelty. The services offered may vary depending on the transition house.

Crisis lines

CRISIS LINES PROVIDE telephone counselling for people in emotional crisis or distress. They may also offer suicide prevention workshops and limited drop-in counselling. You can usually find the telephone number of the crisis line near you in the first few pages of your local telephone book.

Postpartum support organizations

A GROWING NUMBER OF organizations offer support and services to women and families experiencing postpartum depression and anxiety. We recommend that all postpartum support service providers consider becoming members of Postpartum Support International (PSI) and of other national or regional associations. PSI members receive newsletters with information on current issues and relevant publications as well as an annually updated list of member service providers worldwide. Your local health unit may be able to provide you with information on the resources available in your own community The following organizations can also be excellent sources of information and support:

Australia

KARITANE MOTHERCRAFT SOCIETY. Karitane provides a wide variety of services to families, including post natal depression support groups, home visits and residential family care.
PO Box 241, Villawood NSW 2163, AUSTRALIA.
Telephone: (2) 9 794-1800; Fax: (2) 9 794-1858.*

O.P.N.D. (OVERCOMING POST NATAL DISTRESS).
PO Box 306, Daw Park, Adelaide SA 5041, AUSTRALIA.
Telephone: (8) 8 267-1191; Fax: (8) 8 267-3011.*

POST AND ANTE NATAL DEPRESSION ASSOCIATION (PANDA).
PaNDa, Canterbury Family Centre, 19 Canterbury Road, Camberwell VIC 3124, AUSTRALIA.
Telephone: (3) 9 882-5396; Fax: (3) 9 813-3927.*

Canada

PACIFIC POST PARTUM SUPPORT SOCIETY (PPPSS). PPPSS provides support services to women and their families by means of telephone counselling, support groups and literature on PPD. PPPSS also provides information and training to professionals and volunteers. For information on training in group facilitation and telephone support or on services available in B.C., or if you wish to obtain copies of PPPSS publications, contact PPPSS:
#104 - 1416 Commercial Dr., Vancouver BC V5L 3X9, CANADA.
Internet home page: http://www.postpartum.org
Telephone: (604) 255-7999.*

PARENT DEVELOPMENT CENTRE. The Parent Development Centre provides postpartum support.
#405 - 52nd Avenue SW, Calgary AB T2B 0B1, CANADA.
Telephone: (403) 253-8219.*

PASS-CAN, POSTPARTUM ADJUSTMENT SUPPORT SERVICES - CANADA. PASS-CAN is a national organization providing education, direct service and links to other organizations and individuals working in the field of PPD across Canada. PASS-CAN maintains a list of books and videos relevant to PPD.
PO Box 7282, Station Main, Oakville ON L6J 6L6, CANADA.
Telephone: (905) 844-9009; Fax: (905) 844-5973.*

WOMEN'S HEALTH CENTRE AT ST. JOSEPH'S HEALTH CENTRE. The Woman's Health Centre provides postpartum support in English, Polish, Russian, Ukrainian and Spanish.
30 The Queensway, Toronto ON M6R 1B5, CANADA.
Telephone: (416) 530-6850; Fax: (416) 530-6629.*

England

MEET-A-MUM ASSOCIATION (MAMA). MAMA provides a variety of services to women suffering from PPD, including a network of support services and various leaflets and booklets.
MAMA, 14 Willis Road, Croydon SURREY CRO 2XX, ENGLAND.
Telephone: 181 665-0357; Fax: 181 665-1972.*

APNI, ASSOCIATION FOR POST-NATAL ILLNESS. APNI offers telephone support and information to women suffering from PPD by providing information and volunteer telephone support. APNI also raises money to support research on PPD.
APNI, 25 Jerdan Place, Fulham, London SW6 1BE, ENGLAND.
Telephone: 171 386-0868.*

Ireland

POST NATAL DISTRESS ASSOCIATION OF IRELAND.
Carmichael House, North Brunswick St., Dublin 7, IRELAND.
Telephone: 1 872-7172; Fax: 1 873-5737.*

Israel

ISRAEL CHILDBIRTH EDUCATION CENTRE.
Contact: Wendy Blumfield, PO Box 3731, Haifa 31037, ISRAEL.
Telephone: 4 8376820.*

JERUSALEM POSTPARTUM SUPPORT NETWORK.
Contact: Ahava Winston.
PO BOX 292, Telzstone, Harei Yehuda, ISRAEL.
Telephone: 2 533-2810; Fax: 2 533-2811.*

Scotland

THE CHURCH OF SCOTLAND, BOARD OF SOCIAL RESPONSIBILITY: POST-NATAL DEPRESSION PROJECT.
Wallace House, 3 Boswall Rd., Edinburgh Midlothian EH5 3RJ, SCOTLAND.
Telephone: 131 538-7288; Fax: 131 552-2319.*

South Africa

PNDSA — POSTNATAL DEPRESSION SUPPORT ASSOCIATION, SOUTH AFRICA. PNDSA specializes in PPD and offers counselling, assessment, training and conferences.
Contact: Liz Mills, 3 Visser Ave., Trovato Estate,
Kenilworth Cape Town 7700, SOUTH AFRICA.
Telephone: 21 761 5245; Fax: 21 797 4498.*

United States

PSI — POSTPARTUM SUPPORT INTERNATIONAL. PSI is an international organization which maintains a database of member organizations and individuals in the United States and worldwide. This organization provides a variety of services and maintains a list of relevant books and videos. Contact: Jane Honikman. PSI, 927 Kellogg Avenue, Santa Barbara CA 93111, USA.
Email: 74442.3467@compuserve.com; Internet home page: http://www.social.com/health/nhic/data/hr2300/hr2373.html
Telephone: (805) 967-7636; Fax: (805) 967-0608.*

D.A.D. — DEPRESSION AFTER DELIVERY, NATIONAL. D.A.D. is a not-for-profit organization dedicated to providing women with support, information and referrals in matters of postpartum and ante-partum difficulties. D.A.D. keeps a list of members in the United States and Canada and is run mostly by volunteers.
D.A.D., PO Box 1282, Morrisville PA 19067, USA.
Internet home page: http://www.behavenet.com/dadinc
Telephone: 1-(800)-944-4773 or (215) 295-3994.*

International

PSI — POSTPARTUM SUPPORT INTERNATIONAL. PSI maintains a database of member organizations and individuals in the United States and world-wide.
(See listing under the heading "United States".)

MARCÉ SOCIETY is a society of professionals dedicated to improving the understanding, prevention and treatment of mental health problems related to childbearing. This society sponsors international conferences and publishes the *Marcé Bulletin*, which includes articles and summaries on the latest research findings.
The Marcé Society, c/o Dr. Susanne Steinberg (Secretary),
St. Mary's Hospital (Centre hospitalier de St. Mary),
3830 avenue Lacombe, Montréal QC H3T 1M5, CANADA.
Telephone: (514) 345-3511, extension 3851 or 3840;
Fax: (514) 735-1907.*

*** Phone and fax numbers do not include Country codes**

References

1 **PITT, B. (1968).** "'Atypical' depression following childbirth". *British Journal of Psychiatry* 144 (Nov. 1968): 1325-35.

2 **THE BOSTON WOMEN'S HEALTH BOOK COLLECTIVE. (1984).** *The New our bodies, ourselves.* New York: Simon & Schuster.

3 **IBID.**

4 **BARBER, V. & MAGUIRE SKAGGS, M. (1978).** *The mother person.* New York: Schocken Books.

5 **KITZINGER, SHEILA. (1978).** *Women as mothers.* Oxford: Robertson.

About the Pacific Post Partum Support Society

PPPSS IS A NOT-FOR-PROFIT SOCIETY which provides support to women and families experiencing depression or anxiety related to the birth or adoption of a baby. PPPSS also provides training and information for professionals, as well as community education on postpartum depression. The Society publishes *A Self-Help Guide for Mothers* in English and French, as well as *A Group Facilitator's Manual* in English for agencies wishing to facilitate their own support groups.

The philosophy of the Society has always been that the most effective help for postpartum depression and anxiety is non-judgmental support from women who have been through it themselves. The work began in 1971 when a small group of women began meeting to share their experiences and to support each other. This was a new approach to the issue of postpartum depression, and one which has influenced changes in postpartum support worldwide since then.

At PPPSS, we believe that postpartum depression is a family and social issue. Although the PPPSS support groups are for women, telephone support is available for their partners. As well, partners are invited to attend Information Nights to learn more about postpartum depression.

Women who have gone through the groups often say they want to "give something back", and many join the Society as volunteers. Some work in the office, or on special projects. Some join committees or go on the board of directors, and some take training to become telephone support volunteers or group facilitators. All of the Society's staff members and telephone support volunteers are mothers themselves, and they know very well the many joys and stresses of being a parent.

After leaving the groups, women and their partners can also participate in fundraising and publishing activities, and as speakers or facilitators for Information Nights and other outreach events. The participation of committed volunteers greatly extends the range and impact of the services offered by the Pacific Post Partum Support Society.

Our vision is for knowledgeable and caring support to be available for families everywhere, and for awareness about this issue to be so commonplace that the services of the Pacific Post Partum Support Society are no longer necessary.

If you would like to support the Society's work, we invite you to become a Friend of the Society by sending a donation (income tax deductible in Canada) or by leaving a bequest to:

Pacific Post Partum Support Society
1416 Commercial Drive, #104
Vancouver BC V5L 3X9
CANADA

Telephone: (604) 255-7999
Internet home page: http://www.postpartum.org

Federal Tax Exemption #: 10781 0632 RR

A United Way
Affiliate Agency